A Physician's Guide to Therapeutic Massage

John Yates Ph.D.

Curties-Overzet Publications

Many thanks to the following journals for reprint permissions:

Page 20. *JAMA*: Eisenberg D, Davis R, Ettner S, Appel S, Wilkey S, Van Rompay M, Kessler RC. 1998. Trends in Alternative Medicine Use in the United States, 1990-1997. 280:1573, Table 3.

Page 34. *Lymphology*: Yamazaki Z, Fujimori Y, Wada T, Togawa T, Yamakoshi K, Shimazu H. 1979. Admittance plethysmographic evaluation of undulatory massage for the edematous limb. 12:42, Figure 4.

Page 42. *Journal of Gerontology Nursing*: Fakouri C, Jones P. 1987. Relaxation Rx: slow stroke back rub. 13:33, Table 1.

Page 57. *Scandinavian Journal of Rehabilitation Medicine*: Danneskiold-Samsoe B, Christianson E, Lund B, Anderson RB. 1982. Regional muscle tension and pain (fibrositis). Effect of massage on myoglobin in plasma. 15:18, Figure 1.

Page 72. *British Journal of Rheumatology*: Askew LJ, Beckett VL, Kai Nan An, Chao EYS. 1983. Objective evaluation of hand function in scleroderma patients to assess effectiveness of physical therapy. 22:231, Figure 4.

Page 94. *Physical Therapy*: Witt PL, MacKinnon J. 1986. Trager psychophysical integration. A method to improve chest mobility of patients with chronic lung disease. 66:216, Table 3.

A Physician's Guide to Therapeutic Massage
John Yates, Ph.D.

National Library of Canada Cataloguing in Publication

Yates, John, 1945-
A physician's guide to therapeutic massage / John Yates. -- 3rd ed.

Includes bibliographical references and index.
ISBN 0-9685256-4-4

1. Massage therapy. I. Title.

RM721.Y37 2004 615.8'22
C2003-905609-0

To order copies, please contact:
Curties-Overzet Publications Inc.
330 Dupont Street, Suite 400
Toronto, Ontario, Canada M5R 1V9
Toll Free Phone: 1-888-649-5411
Fax: 416-923-8116
Website: www.curties-overzet.com
E-mail: info@curties-overzet.com

Printed and bound in Canada by University of Toronto Press.

Dedication

Have a happy family. And eventually a happy world.

The XIVth Dalai Lama

This book is dedicated to my family, my beloved wife Nancy, my sons John, Charles and Sean, my sisters Claire and Jan, and my parents Bill and Estelle.

It is important not to have the unrealistic expectation
that we will find a magic key to help get rid of all suffering.
It takes determination, patience, and more than one week.

The XIVth Dalai Lama

ACKNOWLEDGEMENTS

Any book is the product of the efforts of many people other than just the author.

I am particularly grateful to Debra Curties for her patience, perseverance and many helpful suggestions throughout the lengthy process of preparing this edition for print. Very special thanks also go to Bev Ransom for her ability to translate thoughts and ideas into brilliant illustrations, and to Tanya-Lynn Paul for her cheerful attitude and efficiency in getting things half-way across the continent as needed and in a timely manner.

I am very much indebted to Trish Dryden, and also to Jean Brown, Peter Becker, Ian Kamm, Lucy Liben, and Dr. Bruce Topp for their time and attention in reading the manuscript, and sincerely appreciate their many useful comments and suggestions. I am also grateful to Dr. Paul Finch for his thoughtful evaluation and comments on the tricky issue of 'older' references.

A very special thank you must also go to my family for their patience, support and encouragement.

Last, but in no way least, I would like to acknowledge my many, many students over the years whose interest and enthusiasm have helped to keep my own alive.

TABLE OF CONTENTS

PREFACE
to the Third Edition

Even as North Americans turn more and more often to massage therapy for help in dealing with stress and to maintain or improve their health, they are also seeking massage treatment with ever greater frequency for injuries and other conditions, both chronic and acute. As a result, physicians are discovering that massage therapy is a useful adjunct to conventional therapy. According to an August 2002 consumer survey commissioned by the American Massage Therapy Association, of the survey respondents who had spoken to their medical doctors about massage therapy, 76% reported that the conversation was favorable.[1] In another survey, 71% of physicians, nurses, and physicians' assistants surveyed in the state of Washington perceived the results of massage therapy as always or usually effective for the purpose it was prescribed.[2]

With this increased interest and demand for integration of massage therapy into mainstream patient care, it is important for physicians to become more knowledgeable about the benefits and efficacy of massage, and about the training and practice standards of massage therapists. The fact is that massage therapy is an economical, low risk, and highly effective form of treatment compared to many other therapies in use today. Well-informed physicians will wish to refer their patients to a massage therapist whose work they know, who is capable, and with whom they can cooperate. Properly trained massage therapists are competent professionals with a potent array of therapeutic techniques at their disposal, and the proficiency to apply them effectively and safely. The physician who makes use of this resource will be able to provide relief for many patients, especially those with musculoskeletal pain and dysfunction.

The views expressed here on the efficacy and safety of massage therapy are the result of twenty years experience working with the profession, fifteen of those years in Vancouver as the Education Director for the West Coast College of Massage Therapy, and also as Research Director for the Massage Therapists Association of British

---

[1] *www.amtamassage.org/infocenter/2002survey.htm*

[2] *Weeks J*, Post-Legislative Mandate: Two Thirds of Group Health Clinician Respondents View CAM as Effective. *The Integrator for the Business of Alternate Medicine, April 2001*

Columbia and consultant to the College of Massage Therapists of British Columbia (the provincial regulatory body) with regard to such issues as curriculum standards for accredited schools and legislative definitions of scope of practice. As the founding President of the Physical Medicine Research Foundation, I have also had the opportunity to explore the complementary roles of orthopedic medicine, sports medicine, physiotherapy, chiropractic, and massage therapy, and to see the development of multi-disciplinary approaches to patient care in practice. For the past six years I have worked with the massage therapy profession in the United States, writing curriculum for schools, developing competencies for the Commission on Massage Therapy Accreditation, planning future initiatives with the National Certification Board for Therapeutic Massage and Bodywork, and as Executive Director of the Council of Massage Therapy Educators in Arizona.

This guide has been written in the hope that, by presenting and advancing the scientific understanding of this remarkable healing technique, it can contribute toward its wider acceptance and utilization by the medical profession. For massage practitioners, a better understanding and greater appreciation of the underlying physiological processes by which their techniques produce the effects they do may pave the way for further refinements in the application of those techniques.

Another intention of this book, in its current as well as previous editions, is to provide a stimulus for further research. Existing research on massage therapy begins to make some progress in demonstrating the nature of its physiological effects on circulation, muscle relaxation, fibrosis, pain, and anxiety. The kneading, 'rubbing,' hacking, and stroking manipulations of Swedish massage, although the most studied to date, represent only a small part of the armamentarium of manual techniques available for use in massage therapy. There remains a genuine need for clinical research into its efficacy in the treatment of specific disorders utilizing all of the powerful techniques that can be incorporated into massage treatment. Also, although manual therapy is widely believed to be most beneficial in the treatment of musculoskeletal pain and dysfunction, this is still not a well researched aspect of massage therapy, an omission that needs to be addressed.

I would like to thank the hundreds of students and practicing massage therapists whose questions over the years have led me to inquire into the physiological basis for the effects that they see on a daily basis.

John Yates, Ph.D.
January, 2004

Passive Movements

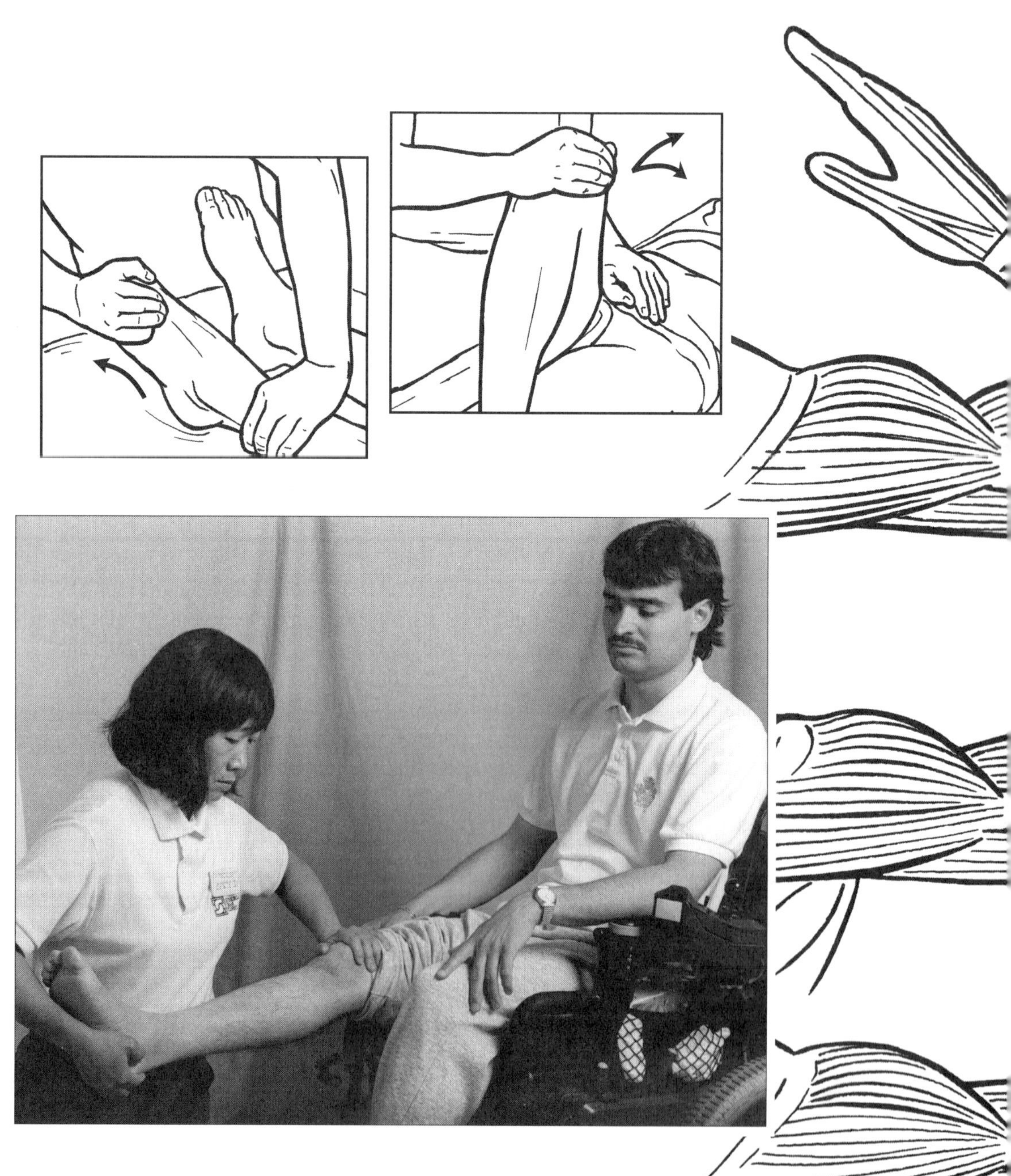

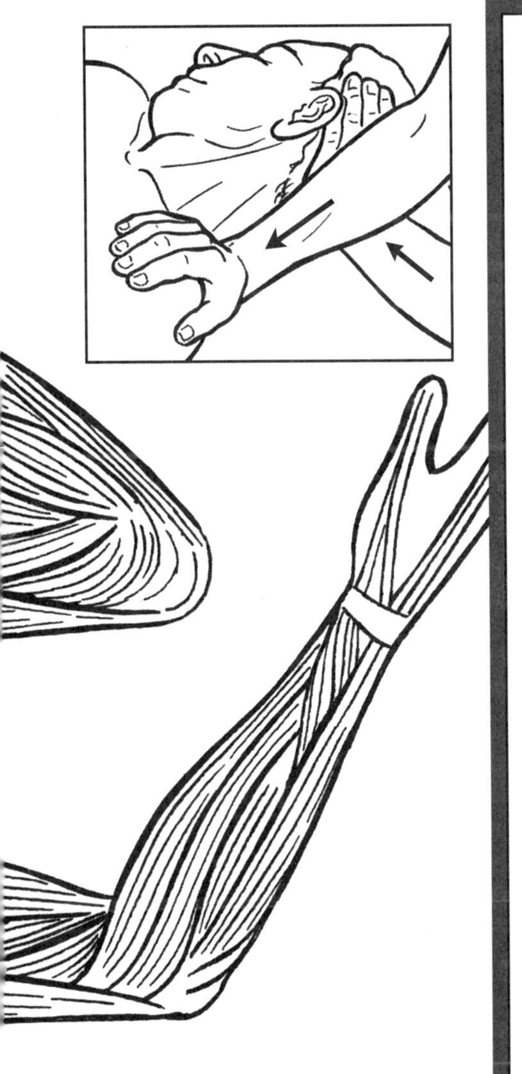

Passive Movements

Passive movements extend from gentle pain free range of motion to forced movements with use of overpressure. Passive movements can also be applied to non-physiological ranges, as in joint play techniques. High velocity thrust techniques are not used.

Customary Uses

- Mobilize tight/stiff joints and connective tissues
- Reflexly decrease muscle tone
- Improve succussive action to rehabilitating or underused joints
- Help align fibers during scar formation, CT rehabilitation
- Reduce psychologically based 'holding' and splinting where appropriate
- Mobilize the thorax and increase ease of breathing
- Facilitate ease of motion/awareness of resistant areas
- Can feel relaxing and nurturing
- Can help prepare for more specific work or bring closure to a body part treatment

Avoid (AV) or Adapt For (AD)

- AV: most acute injuries to bones, soft tissues, blood vessels, nerves
- AV: hemarthrosis, joint mice
- AV: passive forced movement of fragile tendons and joint tissues, bones with severe osteoporosis
- AD: joint and soft tissue inflammatory conditions, joint effusion
- AD: local surgery
- AD: long-term corticosteroid use
- AD: spasticity, rigidity

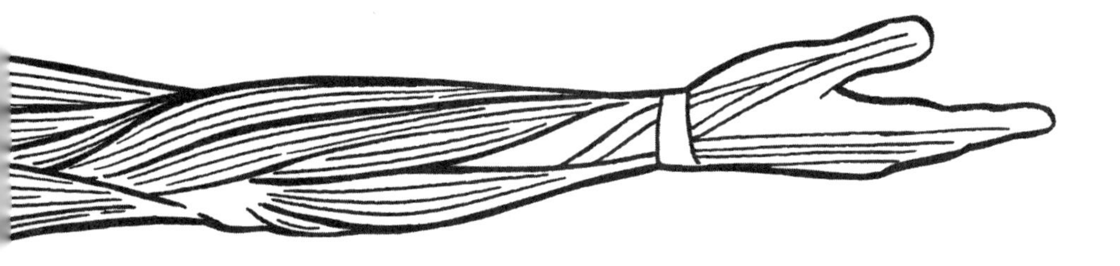

INTRODUCTION

In this age of huge medical research centers, multi-million dollar research budgets for the health sciences, and dramatic pharmacological and technological breakthroughs in the treatment of previously intractable disease, one comes to expect all forms of therapy to rest upon a foundation of scientific and experimental research. In fact, though, much of modern medicine was developed based on principles of treatment that predate this explosive growth in scientific knowledge and health research. These therapeutic principles, the result of an accumulated body of empirical information based on diverse field observation of clinical results, were – and still often are – valid despite the fact that the underlying physiological processes involved have not been studied and elucidated until relatively recently.

This evolution from the empirical to the scientific has been the case with all of the widely accepted conventional forms of treatment. A little more than two decades ago, Wood and Becker (1981:23) recognized that the discipline of massage therapy was undergoing that same transition:

> *Many claims have been made for the use of massage. Some are based upon clinical experience, both objective reports and 'testimonials.' Some are rationalizations of hypotheses based on knowledge of anatomy and physiology. Some are based on controlled, carefully worked out laboratory studies, and some on what might be described as 'wishful thinking.'*

Historically, massage techniques have often been taught by practitioners who lacked adequate training in physiology, pathology, or any of the basic health sciences other than musculoskeletal anatomy. Therefore their students were not trained in these disciplines either. When the need arose to provide a physiological explanation for a technique's beneficial clinical result, the explanation was frequently based on pure – and often inaccurate – conjecture. The appearance of some of these conjectures as statements of fact in manuals of massage therapy has undermined the validity of the treatment in the minds of some people. Nevertheless, just as with medicine in its early days, this therapy's effectiveness in producing positive results has long been evident to its practitioners, their patients, and to the physicians who have made referrals to their services.

Within the last two decades there has been a growing accumulation of scientific evidence that supports and explains the beneficial effects of massage therapy. The significance of this is that increasingly treatment can be prescribed and provided on a scientific rather than an empirical basis. There has also been a significant improvement in both the quantity and quality of basic health sciences education provided to massage therapists.

Massage Techniques

Although many different manual and other techniques are used in massage therapy, only seven major categories of technique are dealt with in the articles reviewed in this guide: Swedish massage, deep friction massage, manual lymph drainage, connective tissue massage, myofascial trigger point therapy, joint mobilization techniques, and therapeutic exercise.

SWEDISH MASSAGE:

Involves palmar, digital, and knuckle movements, including *effleurage* and slow-stroke massage; kneading, rolling, and wringing manipulations, or *petrissage*; frictions (in which the friction occurs between the hand and the subcutaneous tissues); vibration; percussion movements, or *tapotement*; and rhythmic passive movements of joints and body parts.

DEEP FRICTION MASSAGE:

Refers to the specific technique in which the hand remains in contact with the skin and the superficial tissues are moved with respect to the deeper tissues. Dr. James Cyriax is the most widely known proponent of this technique, which is highly specific to the function of disrupting adhesions that have formed or may be forming. Deep friction massage is used for maintaining or restoring painless mobility of musculoskeletal structures. It is considered indispensable in the treatment of many forms of tendinitis.

MANUAL LYMPH DRAINAGE (MLD):

Refers to the specific method developed by Emil and Estrid Vodder for increasing lymphatic flow and clearance to bring about a reduction of tissue fluid accumulation, or edema. It consists of a series of gentle movements of light pressure (approximately 20 to 40 mm Hg), usually applied in a circular pattern, and following the general distribution of lymph vessels draining a body region. This application of light pressure mimics the natural forces moving lymph fluids without disturbing the vascular circulation or triggering histamine release. Although there are a variety of generic lymph drainage massage techniques other than the Vodders', most of the research cited refers to the Vodder method in particular.

CONNECTIVE TISSUE MASSAGE (CTM):

Describes Elisabeth Dicke's technique of applying strokes that produce a tangential pull on the skin to stimulate reflex zones, or connective tissue zones, distributed over the body surface. This technique is considered especially useful in loosening and relaxing tissues preparatory to therapeutic exercises following surgery or trauma, and is claimed to have profound effects on the functioning of the autonomic nervous system. Although the manipulations performed are not unique to CTM, reports that refer specifically to CTM as the intervention under investigation share a greater methodological consistency than do some other studies.

MYOFASCIAL TRIGGER POINT THERAPY:

Involves the systematic location and release of active and latent myofascial trigger points (hyperirritable intramuscular foci) by means of focal deep pressure over the trigger point or a combination of vapocoolant spray and stretching. Trigger point therapy is used to decrease pain on active contraction of affected muscles. It is often applied prior to performing deep tissue massage, joint mobilizations, stretch, or remedial exercise.

JOINT MOBILIZATION TECHNIQUES:

Involve passive movement of a joint beyond the range that can be performed by the patient, either to overcome mechanical resistance or to produce motion in a direction that cannot be produced through voluntary muscle activity. They are used where a restriction exists due to tissue shortening and/or the formation of adhesions within the membranous structures associated with joints, such as occurs with osteoarthritis, traumatic arthritis, meniscal problems, ligamentous sprains, or adhesive capsulitis. The techniques are intended to promote joint nutrition and support restoration of normal range of motion. It should be noted that mobilizations performed by massage therapists do not include the high velocity, low amplitude thrust characteristic of chiropractic manipulations, nor are they used to increase the physiological range of healthy joints.

THERAPEUTIC EXERCISE (OR REMEDIAL EXERCISE):

Refers to the use of corrective exercises in the prevention and treatment of musculoskeletal dysfunction. Such exercises are used to prevent disuse atrophy, adhesions, and contractures, to maintain normal joint range of motion during recovery from injury or disease, and to restore joint and muscle function when these have been compromised. Specific exercises help build muscle strength, endurance and power, improve flexibility and normalize range of motion, and improve coordination, balance, and stability. Therapeutic exercise includes therapist-assisted, therapist-supervised, and home exercise programs.

Manual techniques whose application is not based on a modern Western paradigm have not been considered here. The research cited in this work does not address the effects, therapeutic benefits, or efficacy of touch therapy systems that follow reflexive, energetic, or oriental paradigms of healing.

Standards of Training in Massage Therapy

The education of therapists is certainly relevant to the results that can be expected from treatment. Training, encompassing academic and clinical practicum subject areas, impacts practitioner competency and the efficacy and safety of massage therapy in three areas:

- ability to accurately *assess* the cause of the patient's presenting complaint in order to select and plan appropriate treatment
- capacity to *recognize* conditions for which some therapeutic approaches are contraindicated and to modify treatment accordingly
- mastery of a sufficient variety of soft tissue techniques and other modalities to be able to safely and effectively *perform* the most appropriate form of treatment

The United States lacks uniform national standards for massage therapy training, licensing, and scope of practice. Many states still do not regulate or license massage therapists, and the majority of the states that do so require 500 hours or less of training. The National Certification Board for Therapeutic Massage and Bodywork recognizes a minimum 500-hour training standard, one that is based primarily on hours of instruction and practice without detailed definition of content or competency. On the other hand, the Commission on Massage Therapy Accreditation (COMTA), an accrediting body that has developed both institutional and curriculum standards for massage therapy schools, has introduced a competency based standard that begins to overcome many of these shortcomings. As well, a number of jurisdictions at both the state and municipal level are increasing standards to as much as 1000 hours of training, although definition and standardization of educational content often remain problematic.

In Canada, the provinces of Ontario, Nova Scotia and Newfoundland currently require 2200 hours of training and British Columbia requires 3000 hours. While there is some scope for schools to place their individual stamp on their offerings, the core content of educational programs is mandated by regulatory bodies. Most of the remaining six provinces have an understood 2200-hour requirement without regulation, the driving force usually being the educational hours required as one of the criteria for professional association membership. Alberta and Quebec are exceptions in that the accepted norm for massage therapy education is substantially below 2200 hours.

It is obvious that the same results cannot be expected from a practitioner with 500 hours of training as from one with 2000+ hours. On the other hand, as the information provided in this guide will demonstrate, there is very real benefit to be obtained from referring patients for massage therapy even where local practitioners do not have the highest level of training. Core techniques such as effleurage and slow-stroking massage for improvement of circulation and anxiety reduction, lymph drainage for treatment of edema, and petrissage for muscle tension and soreness are readily mastered at a basic level and are fundamentally safe for most patients (Cherkin et al. 2003; Ernst 2003).

It is also a fact that many of the best documented effects of massage reported in this review are achieved by the application of simple techniques that are not dependent upon extensive training for either effective application or safety of use. Treatment safety on this basis requires that the massage therapist be made aware of circumstances where there are contraindications for the entry level practitioner, such as in the presence of circulatory abnormalities, structural instability, or complex organ system dysfunction. A codified list of contraindications is usually sufficient to prevent harm. One of the most appealing characteristics of massage is that it has stable transitory physiological effects on normal, healthy subjects, and therefore very limited potential to cause injury, while it can have profoundly beneficial effects when properly applied by well-trained practitioners where disorders are present.

Research Literature Review

Chapters 1 through 7 provide a review of readily available and predominantly English language articles in the scientific, medical, and health science literature published between 1885 and 2003. The sources used cover a broad range, including manuals of massage therapy, case reports on the use of massage, articles in nursing journals encouraging the use of massage by hospital nurses, review articles, controlled clinical studies, and experimental research papers on the physiological effects of massage in human and animal subjects.

It was necessary for the organization of this guide to select a set of categories for the various phenomena to be discussed, and inasmuch as this report explores the physiological basis of the effects of massage techniques, an organization based on body systems was chosen. However, while some of the clinical outcomes of massage therapy are clearly the result of effects on specific structures and physiological processes, in many instances it appears that they are products of a complex interaction of several mechanisms including mechanical, neural, chemical, and psychological factors.

Accordingly, the more non-specific effects of massage have been grouped together in Chapter 1, and the physiological effects that can be more readily identified with specific functional systems have been organized into separate topics on that basis in Chapters 2 through 7. These topics are: the circulation of blood and lymph, the processes of fibrosis and repair, functional effects upon the musculature, the control of pain, respiratory function, and the psychoemotional status of the individual.

A list of conditions where therapeutic massage is indicated has been provided at the end of each section. Although many of these pathologies involve more than one body system, they are categorized under specific body systems for the sake of presentation. In practice, appropriate massage techniques are matched to specific treatment goals. In some cases the treatment goal deals directly with the problem body system, such as, for example, improved circulation in a patient with varicose veins. In another situation the treatment goal may focus on a system that will indirectly encourage the rehabilitation of a lesion in another body system, as in the case of increasing circulation in the treatment of supraspinatus tendinitis.

It is notable that, by and large, only the simplest techniques and effects have been investigated so far. Many of the circulatory and anxiety reduction benefits reported in this review were achieved by the application of basic stroking and kneading techniques, and in the case of some circulatory effects, were even performed by mechanical devices. As the research cited here demonstrates, the mechanisms by which massage therapy techniques can be expected to produce beneficial therapeutic results have been reasonably well studied. What is particularly lacking is research on the clinical efficacy of the range of massage therapy techniques when utilized as part of a coherent therapeutic system by therapists with extensive training in clinical assessment and treatment planning. For example, literature reviews of clinical research on massage therapy for the treatment of low back pain by Ernst in 1999 and Furlan et al. in 2000 concluded that high quality clinical trials were needed before the value of massage for back pain could be determined. Although a similar review by Cherkin et al. in 2003 identified three new studies on back pain, massage therapy efficacy in addressing the full range of musculoskeletal injuries and dysfunctions remains relatively unstudied. This promises to be a very fruitful area for future investigations.

Swedish Massage Technique Stroking

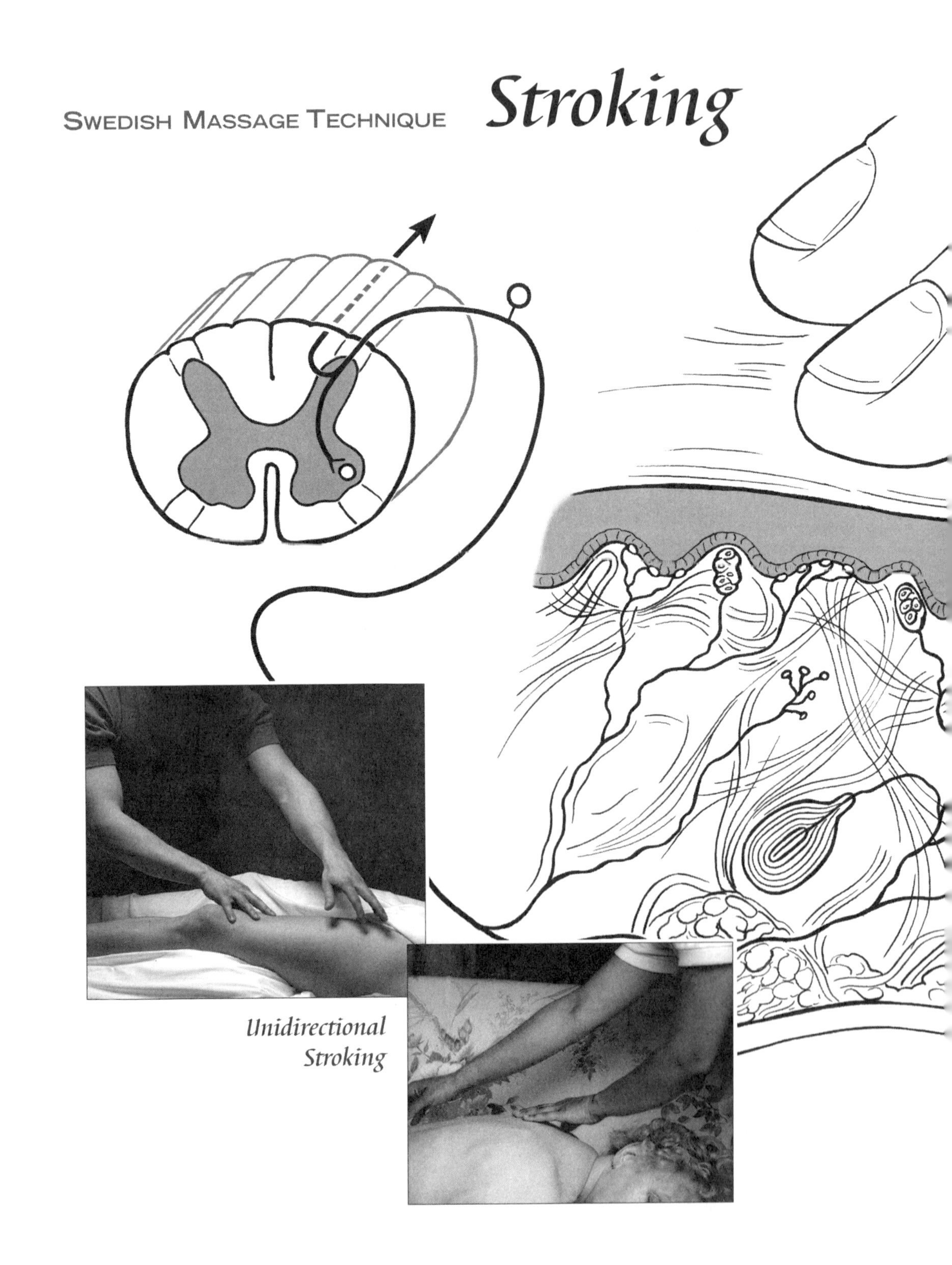

Unidirectional Stroking

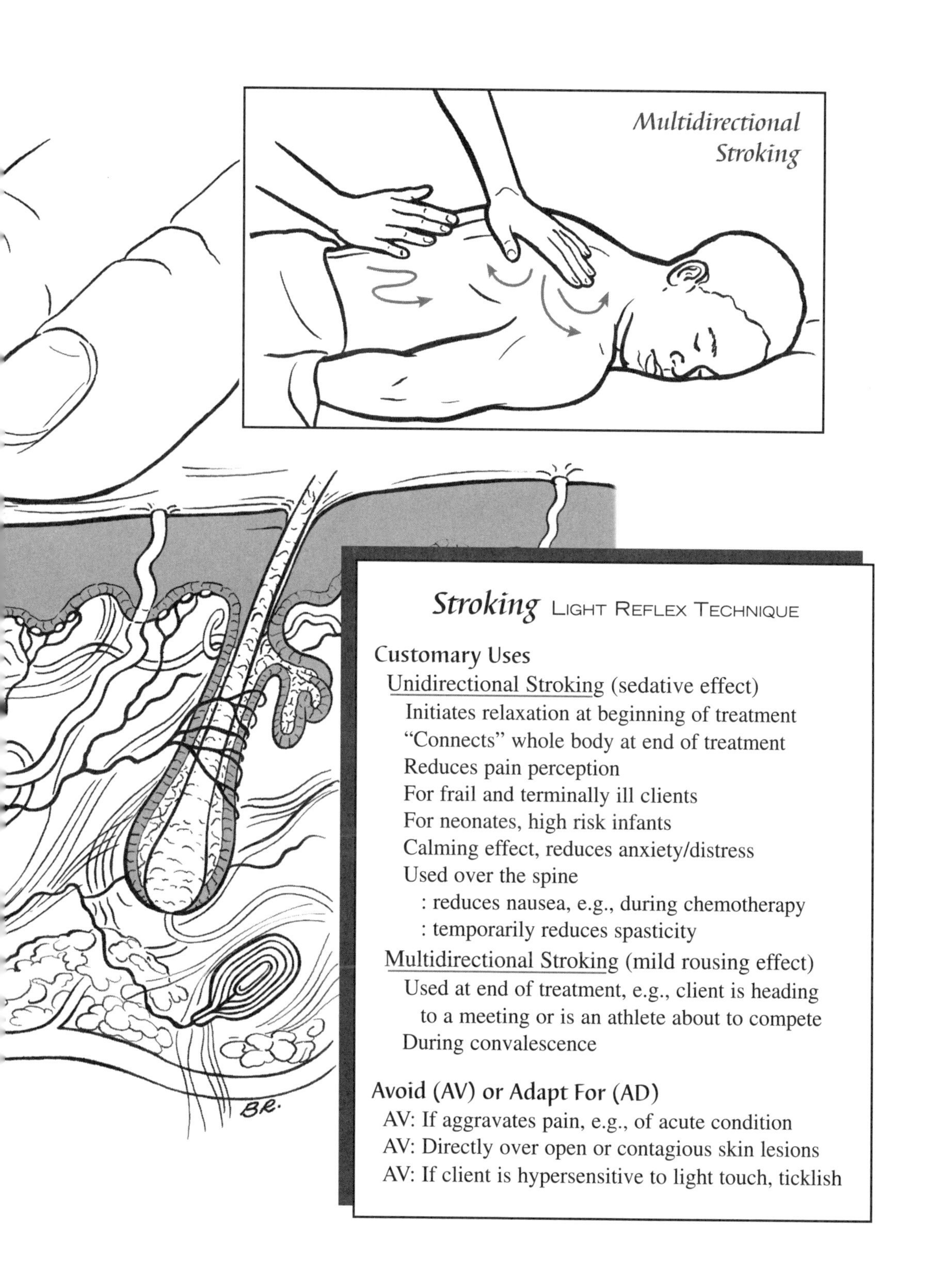

Stroking Light Reflex Technique

Customary Uses

<u>Unidirectional Stroking</u> (sedative effect)

- Initiates relaxation at beginning of treatment
- "Connects" whole body at end of treatment
- Reduces pain perception
- For frail and terminally ill clients
- For neonates, high risk infants
- Calming effect, reduces anxiety/distress
- Used over the spine
  - : reduces nausea, e.g., during chemotherapy
  - : temporarily reduces spasticity

<u>Multidirectional Stroking</u> (mild rousing effect)

- Used at end of treatment, e.g., client is heading to a meeting or is an athlete about to compete
- During convalescence

Avoid (AV) or Adapt For (AD)

AV: If aggravates pain, e.g., of acute condition
AV: Directly over open or contagious skin lesions
AV: If client is hypersensitive to light touch, ticklish

1 Understanding the Scope of Application of Therapeutic Massage: The Wellness Model

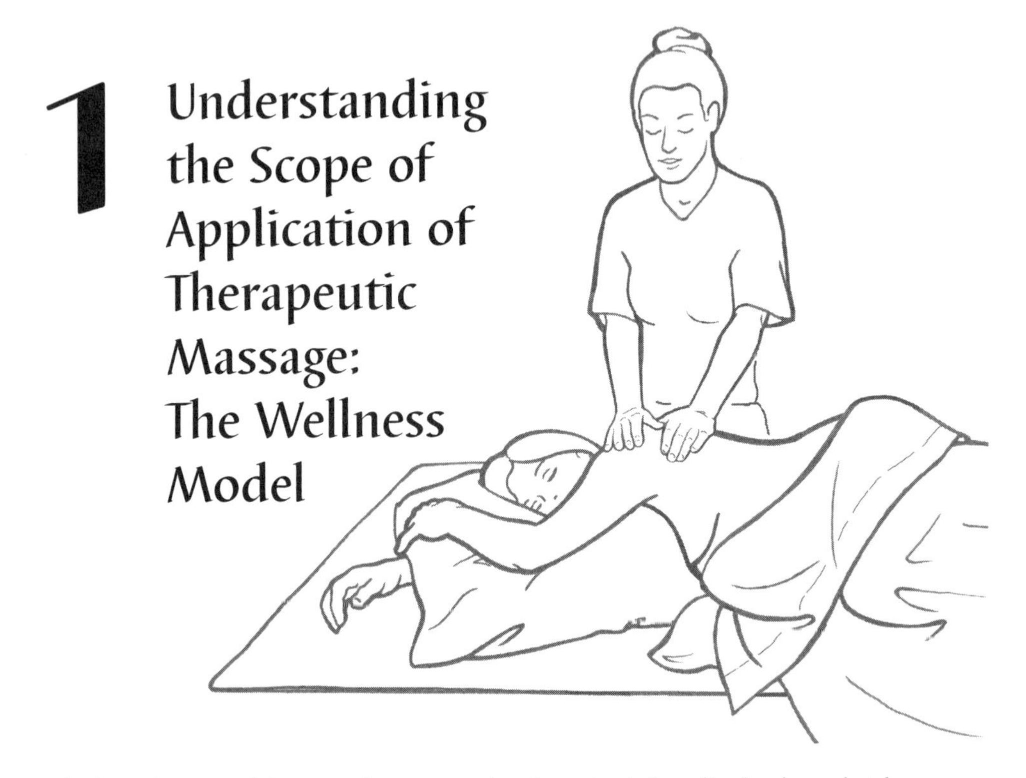

The broad scope of therapeutic massage has been best described using what has come to be known as the "wellness model" (Tappan & Benjamin, 1998, pg 3-10). The wellness model may be visualized as a degrees of health continuum extending from premature death at one extreme to high-level wellness at the other. In the middle is a "neutral point" characterized by the absence of either discernible illness or robust health. Between the extreme of premature death and the neutral point is a region where impairment and/or signs and symptoms of disease are evident. Conventional medical practice is usually focused on and operates within this region of the continuum, constituting what has been described as a "treatment model." The focal points in the treatment model are diagnosis and treatment of the condition responsible for illness; treatment is typically discontinued shortly after the neutral point has been achieved.

The intent of the practitioner operating within the wellness model is to help recipients of treatment to attain increased well-being, regardless of where they are on the continuum at the time of treatment. In the presence of overt disease or injury, the general intent is to help the patient/client achieve improved wellness within the constraints imposed by the condition. When the recipients of treatment are free of disease and injury, the general intent is to help them attain higher level wellness, moving further toward optimal well-being.

Whatever the health status of the client, the wellness approach encompasses a holistic view of people as physical, emotional, intellectual, social, and spiritual beings. From this holistic perspective, skilled touch has the possibility to influence recipients across all spheres, and massage therapists practice in the belief that skilled, caring touch promotes health at many different levels regardless of the presence or absence of medical conditions.

Using the wellness model and regarding the treatment paradigm as a subset of this model, two different aspects of intention can be distinguished in the approach to treatment – treatment to promote wellness in a general sense, and treatment to bring about specific therapeutic effects. Treatment for general therapeutic benefit has as its primary focus the improvement of the sense of well-being and overall wellness of the individual, and is not primarily directed toward the alleviation of specific signs and symptoms or the underlying pathological mechanisms that are responsible for them. Treatment for specific therapeutic benefit, by contrast, is directed precisely at the underlying pathology and/or presenting symptomatology.

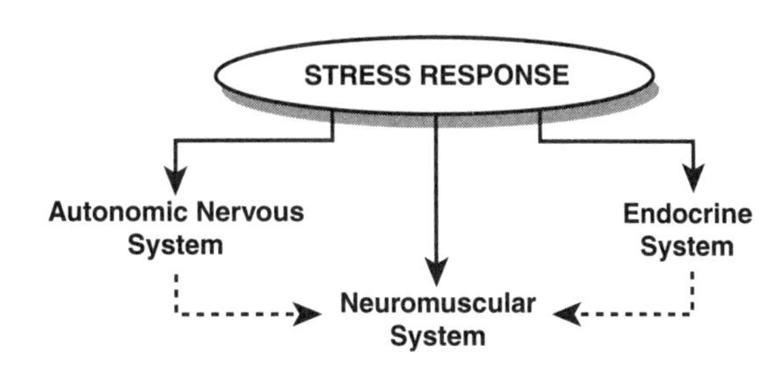

General therapeutic benefits of massage therapy help the recipient move closer to optimal well-being by creating positive outcomes in that person's life. Mental and physical relaxation, improved circulation, enhanced energy and vitality, symptomatic relief of excessive muscle tone and other non-specific musculoskeletal aches and pains, greater flexibility and range of motion, psychological stress and anxiety reduction, self acceptance, and experiencing comfort through touch are examples of general therapeutic benefits of massage and bodywork. The most commonly sought therapeutic benefit of massage is the relief of discomfort brought on by stress and chronic muscular tension.

To date, it is accurate to say that most massage practitioners in the United States function largely within the scope of promoting general therapeutic benefits. From this perspective, it can be seen that a person with a specific injury or condition may receive massage treatment for its general therapeutic benefits and not necessarily to address the pathology directly. Nevertheless, the general therapeutic benefits of massage may have a positive effect on a problem condition, even where this is not the primary intention of treatment. In either case, the recipient is closer to a state of optimal well-being.

Massage therapy may, of course, also be used with specific therapeutic intent. This treatment paradigm is sometimes referred to as "medical massage," and it is the predominant practice model of massage therapy in Canada and European countries. In British Columbia, for example, massage therapy is fully accepted as part of the health care system, and approximately 70% of patients treated by massage therapists do so on referral from a physician.[1] Also, once their preliminary evaluation has indicated that referral to a massage therapist is appropriate, general practice physicians commonly rely upon the massage therapist to perform an assessment and devise an appropriate treatment plan. The College of Massage Therapists of BC has estimated that only about 5% of physician referrals state a specific diagnosis.

Table 3.—Comparison of Use of Alternative Therapies for the Most Frequently Reported Principal Medical Conditions, 1997 vs 1990

	Percentage Reporting Condition		Used Alternative Therapy for Condition in Past 12 mo, %		Saw Alternative Practitioner for Condition in Past 12 mo, %		Saw Medical Doctor and Used Alternative Therapy for Condition in Past 12 mo, %		Saw Medical Doctor and Alternative Practitioner for Condition in Past 12 mo, %		
Condition	**1997**	**1990**	**1997**	**1990**	**1997**	**1990**	**1997**	**1990**	**1997**	**1990**	**Therapies Most Commonly Used in 1997**
Back problems	24.0#	19.9	47.6#	35.9	30.1#	19.5	58.8**	36.1	39.1#	23.0	Chiropractic, massage
Allergies	20.7#	16.0	16.6#	8.7	4.2	3.3	28.0¶	15.7	6.4	5.0	Herbal, relaxation
Fatigue*	16.7	...	27.0	...	6.3	...	51.6	...	13.1	...	Relaxation, massage
Arthritis	16.6	15.9	26.7¶	17.5	10.0	7.8	38.6¶	23.8	15.9	13.8	Relaxation, chiropractic
Headaches	12.9	13.2	32.2	26.5	13.3¶	6.3	42.0	31.8	20.0	12.1	Relaxation, chiropractic
Neck problems*	12.1	...	57.0	...	37.5	...	66.6	...	47.5	...	Chiropractic, massage
High blood pressure	10.9	11.0	11.7	11.0	0.9	2.9	11.9	11.6	1.1	3.5	Megavitamins, relaxation
Sprains or strains	10.8	13.4	23.6	22.3	10.3	9.6	29.4	24.7	15.9	13.6	Chiropractic, relaxation
Insomnia	9.3#	13.6	26.4	20.4	7.6	4.0	48.4	19.8	13.3	10.9	Relaxation, herbal
Lung problems	8.7	7.3	13.2	8.8	2.5	0.5	17.9	11.1	3.4	0.6	Relaxation, spiritual healing, herbal
Skin problems	8.6	8.0	6.7	6.0	2.2	1.6	6.8	6.9	0.0	2.5	Imagery, energy healing
Digestive problems	8.2	10.1	27.3#	13.2	9.7¶	3.6	34.1¶	15.3	10.7	5.8	Relaxation, herbal
Depression†	5.6	8.4	40.9	20.2	15.6	7.0	40.9	35.2	26.9	14.0	Relaxation, spiritual healing
Anxiety‡	5.5	9.5	42.7	27.9	11.6	6.5	42.7	45.4	21.0	10.4	Relaxation, spiritual healing
Weighted average across all conditions§	...	...	28.2**	19.1	11.4**	6.8	31.8**	19.9	13.7#	8.3	...
People with ≥1 condition‖	77.8¶	81.5	33.7**	22.9	15.3**	6.9	...	...	...	...	...

*Not included as a separate question in 1990 survey. Ellipses indicate data not applicable.
†The 1997 question asked about severe depression, which is not directly comparable with the 1990 question that asked about depression.
‡The 1997 question asked about anxiety attacks, which is not directly comparable with the 1990 question that asked about anxiety.
§The weighted averages are calculated based on all 37 conditions studied in 1997 and all 24 conditions studied in 1990, ie, condition is unit of analysis.
‖This row shows percentage of respondents who reported 1 or more principal medical conditions, along with the percentage of these respondents who reported use of therapy or practitioners for at least 1 of these conditions, ie, person is the unit of analysis.
¶$P \le .05$; #$P \le .01$; **$P < .001$.

Eisenberg DM, et al. Trends in Alternative Medicine Use in the United States, 1990-1997, *JAMA 1998; 280:1573.*

The majority of U.S. massage practitioners would require extensive post-graduate training in order to be able to function independently within a specific treatment model. Nevertheless, the current level of training and competency of American massage

[1] *Statistics provided by the College of Massage Therapists of British Columbia*

therapists in basic manual techniques is more than adequate to provide the majority of the therapeutic benefits described in this guide upon referral and with minimal input from the primary care physician. As well, a number of U.S. practitioners do have post-graduate training that greatly adds to their expertise in specific condition-based treatment.

The only *caveat* to the foregoing is with regard to the conditions and treatment modalities discussed in Chapters 3 and 4. Therapeutic stretch, joint mobilizations, fascial mobilization, and deep friction massage are part of an array of powerful manual therapeutic techniques that can be used in the treatment of more serious musculoskeletal dysfunctions. They can be profoundly effective for certain conditions, but they do require more skill and training to apply effectively as there is the potential for exacerbating existing injury or causing new injury. As well, their application requires the assessment capability to determine their appropriateness and to adapt treatment to the current state of the involved tissue. Attempts to use these techniques without adequate training are at best ineffective and at worst potentially harmful. At present, these more advanced techniques represent an extremely valuable and very much underutilized contribution of manual therapy to health care, particularly in the U.S.

It is hoped that the information provided in this guide will contribute to the development of improved definitions and standards for the licensing of massage therapists and accreditation of massage therapy training programs in jurisdictions throughout North America and elsewhere. If so, the public will benefit from access to many more well trained massage therapists than are now available, and I believe that this will be positively received by physicians and medical insurers as well.

General Benefits of Massage: Psychological and Behavioral

The non-specific therapeutic benefits that have been demonstrated include psychological and behavioral parameters such as:

- improved mood
- reduced anxiety
- lower stress levels
- lessening of depression
- reduced anger and aggression
- improved sleep patterns and decreased sleep disturbance

ANXIETY AND STRESS are found to be reduced in children with diabetes (Field 1998; Field et al. 1997e; Field 1995), juvenile RA (Field et al. 1997a; Field 1995), and PTSD (Field 1998; Field et al. 1996b; Field 1995); in back pain (Hernandez-Reif et al. 2001b; Hernandez-Reif et al. 2000a), cancer (Billhult & Dahlberg 2001; Stephenson et al. 2000; Burke et al. 1994), burn (Field et al. 1998a or 1997h) and post-burn (Field et al. 2000), chronic fatigue syndrome (CFS) (Field et al. 1997f), fibromyalgia (Field et al. 2002; Sunshine et al. 1996), HIV positive (Diego et al. 2001; Ironson et al. 1996), multiple sclerosis (Hernandez-Reif et al. 1998b), and sexual abuse patients (Field et al. 1997d; Field 1995); during pregnancy (Field et al. 1999), labor and delivery (Field et al. 1997c); and in individuals experiencing job stress (Field et al. 1997g; Field et al. 1996a), and premenstrual symptoms (Hernandez-Reif et al. 2000b).

Massage is effective as a stress reducer for psychiatric in- and out-patients (Hilliard 1995), in diffusing agitated behaviors in individuals with Alzheimer's Disease (Rowe & Alfred 1999), and in relieving anxiety/relaxing long-term terminal care and hospice patients (Hemphill & Kemp 2000; Dawson & Kontos 1998; Urba 1996; Bumpus 1993; Meck 1993).

Symptoms of distress are also shown to be reduced during treatment of child burn victims (Hernandez-Reif et al. 2001a; Field 1998, 1995), in migraine sufferers (Hernandez-Reif et al. 1998a), in cocaine exposed and intensive care neonates (Scafidi et al. 1996; Field 1995; Wheeden et al. 1993; Field 1992), and in infants of depressed mothers (Field et al. 1996d; Field 1995). Subjective reports and observations of reduced anxiety and stress following massage have been demonstrated in many cases to be correlated with objective indicators such as reduced stress hormone levels (cortisol and norepinephrine), lowered pulse rate, and decreased diastolic blood pressure.

DEPRESSION has been reported to be decreased in children with diabetes (Field 1998; Field et al. 1997e; Field 1995) and PTSD (Field 1998; Field et al. 1996b; Field 1995); in juvenile and adolescent psychiatric patients (Field et al. 1992); in anorexia (Hart et al. 2001), bulimia (Field et al. 1997b), back pain (Hernandez-Reif et al. 2001b, 2000a), breast cancer (Stephenson et al. 2000), burn (Field et al. 1998a, 1997h), CFS (Field et al. 1997f), fibromyalgia (Field et al. 2002; Sunshine et al. 1996), MS (Hernandez-Reif et al. 1998b), HIV positive (Diego et al. 2001), and sexual abuse patients (Field et al. 1997d); post-partum (Onozawa et al. 2001), and in teenage mothers (Jones & Field 1999; Field et al. 1996c); and in individuals experiencing job stress (Field et al. 1997g; Field et al. 1996a). These subjectively reported and observed changes have likewise been correlated with such objective indicators as increased serotonin and dopamine levels and attenuation of right frontal EEG asymmetry, a pattern associated with depression.

ANGER was found to be decreased by massage therapy in burn and post-burn patients (Field et al. 2000; Field et al. 1998a, 1997h). Bulimics and anorexics were found to have an improved body image and decreased body dissatisfaction (Hart et al. 2001; Field et al. 1997b). There is a case report of massage producing a beneficial effect on self-injury behavior in Cornelia de Lange Syndrome (Dossetor et al. 1991). Massage treatment for adolescents with ADHD resulted in less fidgeting and greater self-rated happiness (Abrams 2000; Field et al. 1998c). Autistic children treated with massage therapy have been found to have decreased off-task classroom behavior, improved "relatedness" to teachers, increased attentiveness and responsivity, and decreased touch sensitivity (Field et al. 1997h). Children with diabetes have also been found to show improved dietary compliance with regular massage (Field et al. 1997e).

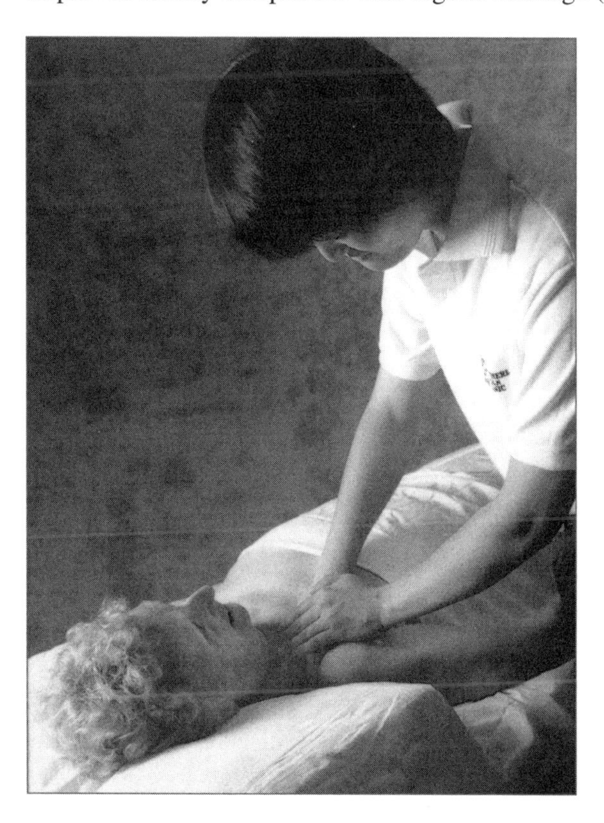

IMPROVED SLEEP PATTERNS have been found to occur following regular massage in preterm neonates and infants with sleep disturbances (Field & Hernandez-Reif 2001; Field et al. 1996c; Scafidi et al. 1986), autistic children (Escalona et al. 2001), preschool children (Field et al. 1996e), adolescent psychiatric patients (Field et al. 1992), pregnant women (Field et al. 1999), the critically ill (Culpepper-Richards 1998) and terminal care patients (Urba 1996), and in patients with back pain (Hernandez-Reif et al. 2001b; Hernandez-Reif et al. 2000a), CFS (Field et al. 1997f), fibromyalgia (Sunshine et al. 1996), Parkinson's Disease (Hernandez-Reif et al. 2002), and migraine sufferers (Hernandez-Reif et al. 1998a).

A more detailed discussion of some of these studies with reference to the benefits of massage therapy in relieving anxiety and depression is provided in Chapter 7, which specifically addresses psychological effects.

The treatment protocols in the studies mentioned in this chapter most commonly consist of simple stroking and kneading in the form of back, or sometimes foot, massages for 15 to 30 minutes at a time. Typical treatment frequency is twice per week, and outcomes are usually determined between two weeks and one month after the beginning of the treatment program. Although the authors cited here have not demonstrated it to be so, the impression given by such consistency in methodology is that the findings reflect the cumulative result of a treatment series that is most evident following four to eight sessions. The effects appear to be primarily the result of an experience of "caring touch," a soothing and/or pleasurable tactile stimulation performed in a non-threatening environment within an emotional atmosphere of giving and caring.

The simplest and therefore most likely explanation is that massage treatment is activating a powerful innate psychobiological response related to touch.

Although it is possible that the effects outlined here are mediated by subtle mechanisms that have yet to be identified, the simplest and therefore most likely explanation is that massage treatment is activating a powerful innate psychobiological response related to touch. The numerous beneficial responses to massage in infants and neonates (described below) are consistent with this view. Improvements in affective state and perceived stress along with associated endocrine and neurohormonal changes may be hypothesized as the primary psychobiological response.

Other General Therapeutic Benefits of Massage

There are numerous other positive therapeutic effects that are probably secondary to or closely related to changes in mood, reductions in anxiety, depression, and perceived stress, and improvements in relaxation and subjective well-being. These include enhanced cognitive behavior, reduced fatigue, improved immune system function, increased peak air flow in asthmatics (Field et al. 1998b) and children with cystic fibrosis (Hernandez-Reif et al. 1999), lowered blood glucose in diabetic children (Field et al. 1997e; Field 1995), decreased frequency of occurrence of migraine headaches (Hernandez-Reif et al. 1998a), decreased pain perception, and improved functional abilities in patients with spinal cord injury (Diego et al. 2002). Decreased white blood cell and neutrophil counts in children with leukemia (Field et al. 2001) appear to belong in this category as well.

Massage has been found to enhance learning behaviors in infants (Cigales et al. 1997), and to improve COGNITIVE PERFORMANCE in preschool children (Hart et al. 1998). It also resulted in adults being able to complete math problems in less time with fewer errors; they demonstrated decreased frontal EEG alpha and beta waves and increased delta activity consistent with enhanced alertness (Field et al. 1996a).

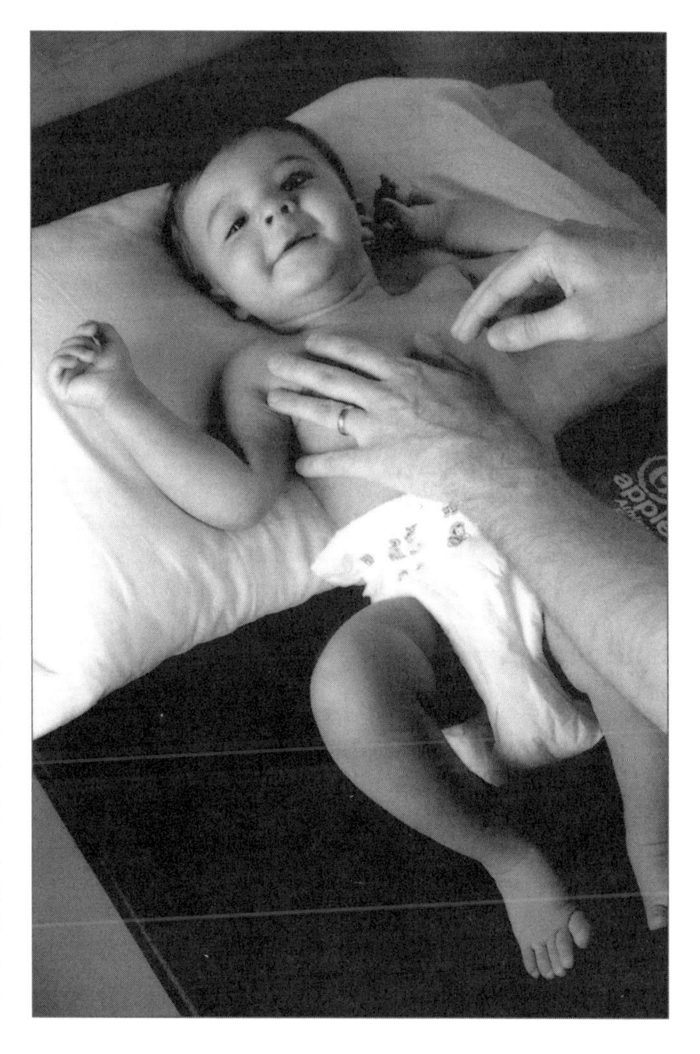

Reduced FATIGUE has been reported in individuals treated by massage for fibromyalgia (Offenbacher & Stucki 2000; Sunshine et al. 1996), job stress (Field et al. 1997g; Field et al. 1996a), CFS (Field et al. 1997f), and in caregivers of patients undergoing stem cell transplant (Rexilius et al. 2002).

IMMUNE FUNCTION improvement following massage treatment, as indicated by increased natural killer cell number, increased CD4 cells, and increased CD4/CD8 ratio, has been documented for healthy students (Zeitlin et al. 2000) and HIV positive adults and adolescents (Diego et al 2001; Ironson et al. 1996).

In addition to the specific physiological mechanisms by which massage therapy directly impacts on pain (discussed in Chapter 5), massage has also been reported to have a beneficial effect on PAIN PERCEPTION (Mobily et al. 1994) in a wide variety of conditions. Following a regular program of massage, individuals with juvenile RA (Field et al. 1997a), burns (Field et al. 2000, 1998a, 1997h), cancer (Stephenson et al. 2000; Grealish et al. 2000; Wilkie et al. 2000; Ferrell-Torry & Glick 1993), CFS (Field et al. 1997f; Kantrowitz et al. 1995), fibromyalgia (Offenbacher & Stucki 2000; Sunshine et al. 1996), and premenstrual symptoms (Hernandez-Reif et al. 2000b), as well as terminal care patients (Urba 1996) and HIV positive individuals with severe neuropathy (Acosta et al. 1998) all reported experiencing less pain. Studies of patients with back pain have provided mixed results, with some reports of improvement and others suggesting not (Cherkin et al. 2001; Hernandez-Reif et al. 2001b; Furlan et al. 2000; Preyde 2000; Hernandez-Reif et al. 2000a; Ernst 1999; Pope et al. 1994; Gibson 1988).

In addition to the specific physiological mechanisms by which massage therapy directly impacts on pain, massage has also been reported to have a beneficial effect on pain perception.

Massage has been found to reduce pain for women in labor (Field et al. 1997c). Massage in pregnancy and during labor has also been shown to be associated with decreased obstetric complications, lower prematurity rates, shorter labor, shorter hospital stays, and decreased depression following birth (Field et al. 1999, 1997c).

Neonates and Infants

Massage has been observed to alleviate stress in intensive care (Field 1990, 1987), and cocaine exposed (Wheeden et al. 2000) neonates, as evidenced by fewer startle responses and other stress behaviors like grimacing and clenched fists. Massaged preterm infants have been shown to have decreased plasma cortisol levels (Acolet et al. 1993), and were also observed to be more socially responsive (Field et al. 1986). Infants of depressed mothers displayed less fussiness, improved sociability and soothability, and improved interaction behaviors; these changes were associated with lower cortisol and norepinephrine and increased serotonin levels (Field et al. 1996d).

Intensive care (Field 1990), preterm (Ferber et al. 2002; Scafidi et al. 1986), HIV exposed (Scafidi & Field 1997), and cocaine exposed (Scafidi et al. 1996) neonates and infants of depressed mothers (Field et al. 1996d) all showed greater weight gain with massage. These studies also found that massaged intensive care, HIV exposed, and cocaine exposed neonates scored better on the Brazelton Scale. Cocaine exposed and intensive care neonates had fewer postnatal complications, intensive care neonates had decreased need for ventilation, and preterm neonates were discharged six days earlier and showed more optimal cognitive and motor development eight months later.

Conclusions and Application

Changes such as those demonstrated in behavioral factors and sleep patterns likely flow from improved neurobiological status in the organism as a whole. Put most simply, massage makes people feel better, and there appears to be an across-the-board improvement in physiological function when people feel better. It is significant about the research presented here that there is consistent intervention simplicity as well as efficacy of results across the complete spectrum of age and health status.

> *Massage is indicated as a valuable complement reinforcing and increasing the effectiveness of other forms of treatment for a large variety of conditions, indeed including almost any condition for which medical treatment may be sought.*

Massage is indicated as a valuable complement reinforcing and increasing the effectiveness of other forms of treatment for a large variety of conditions, indeed including almost any condition for which medical treatment may be sought. This is most particularly true where response to treatment is less than expected (e.g. impaired immunity), where increased medication is contraindicated or ineffective (e.g. analgesic narcotics), or where decreases in medication may be desirable (e.g. psychotropic drugs). Also, a prescription for training of parents in the techniques of infant and child massage may be a highly cost effective approach to improved management of a whole range of pediatric issues and conditions.

Effleurage

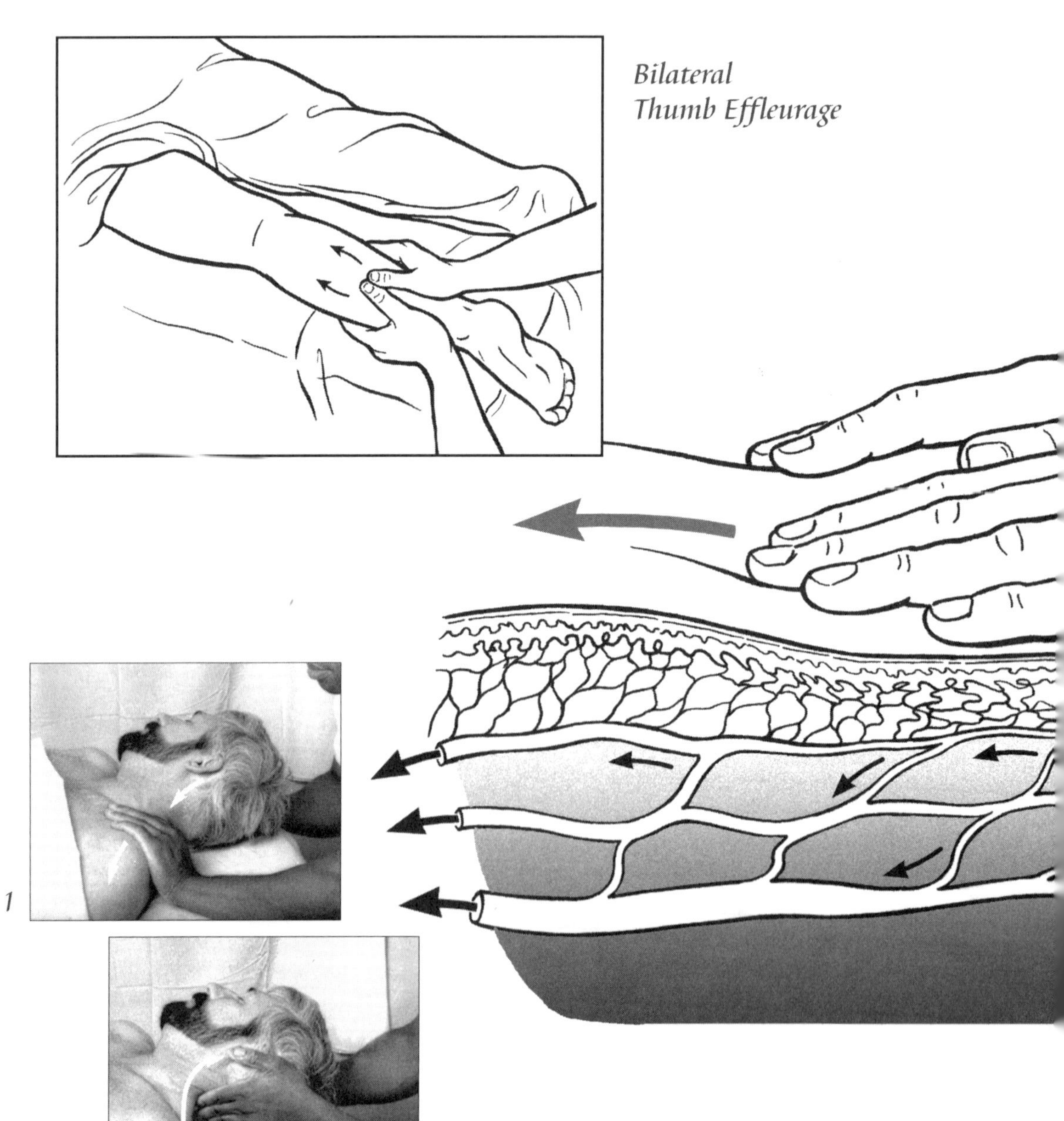

Bilateral Thumb Effleurage

1

2

Neck Effleurage Sequence

Back Effleurage Sequence

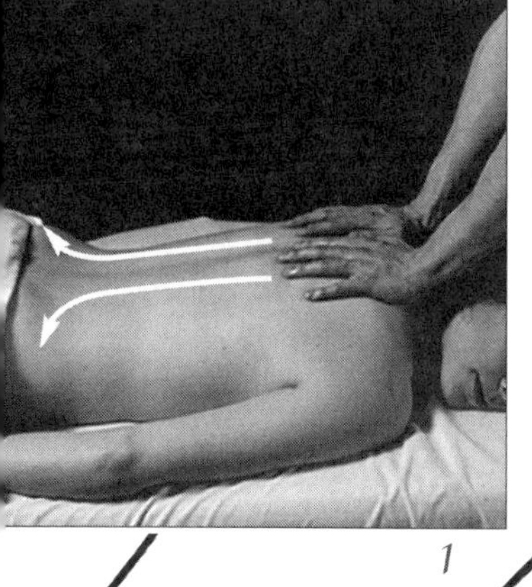
1

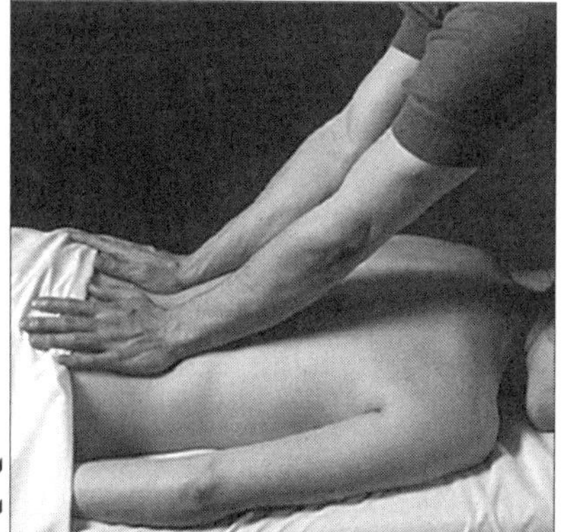
2

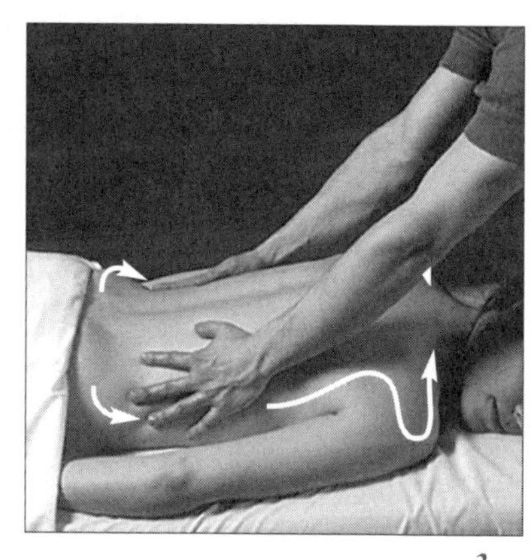
3

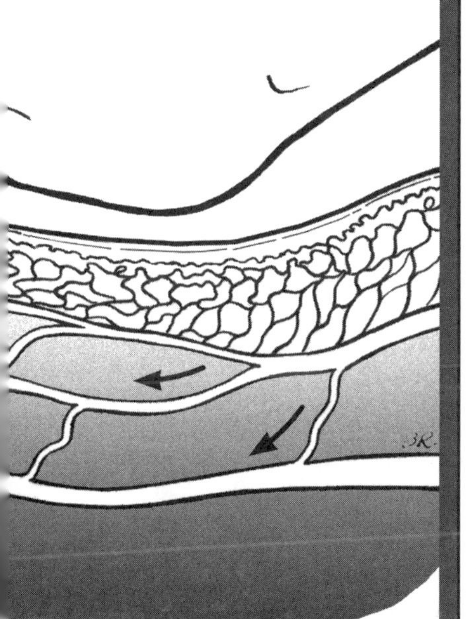

Effleurage GLIDING FLUID MOBILIZER

Customary Uses

Spreads lubricant and introduces therapist's touch
Preparation for more specific work; transition stroke
Mobilizes venous return and lymph drainage from treated body part to core circulation
Reduces congestion and edema
Reduces lower motor neuron excitability
Stimulates peristalsis
When applied lightly, has sedative and analgesic effects similar to unidirectional stroking
When applied deeply, engages fascia and muscle tissues similar to broad petrissage

Avoid (AV) or Adapt For (AD)

AV: Contagious lesions, early stage healing, sepsis
AD: Proximal only to contusions, inflamed tissue
AD: Reflex sympathetic dystrophy
AV: Phlebitis, phlebothrombosis
AD: Hypertension, congestive heart failure
AD: Wait 48 hours following coronary bypass
AV: Very diseased/degenerative kidneys

2 Circulation of Blood and Lymph

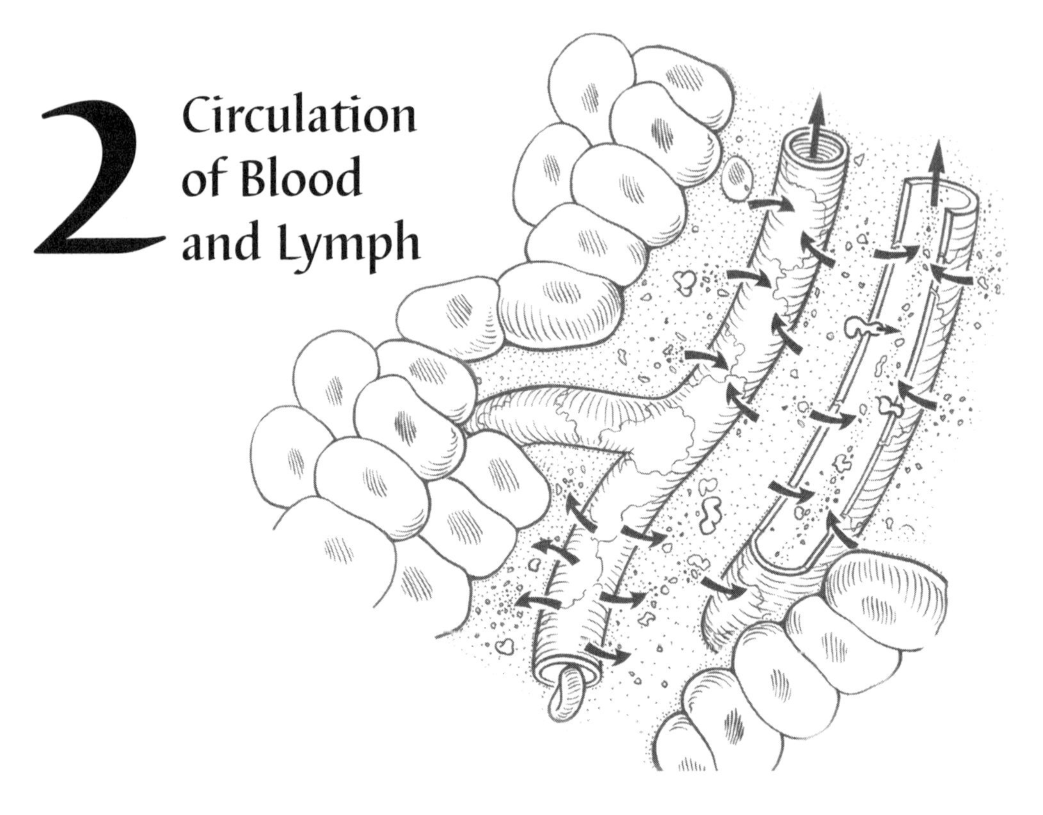

Increases in the blood and lymph circulation (Wale 1968) are the most widely recognized and frequently described of the physiological effects of massage therapy. Changes in blood and lymph circulation are appropriately discussed together because they have effects in common on the clearance of metabolic wastes and by-products of tissue damage and inflammation, the absorption of excess inflammatory exudate, and on the delivery of oxygen and nutrients to tissue cells.

Removal of waste materials can be accomplished by an increase in blood flow through the capillaries or via an increased rate of lymph formation. Lymph removal through lymphatic capillaries and vessels brings about a flushing of the interstitial fluid along with macromolecular and particulate materials.

As well, both the vascular and the lymphatic circulations influence effective delivery of oxygen and nutrients to cells. Blood circulation maintains a sufficient capillary concentration to create a gradient that enables diffusion of oxygen and nutrients to the cells. The lymph circulation, in contrast, determines the relative degree of accumulation or removal of interstitial fluid and thereby affects the distance over which these essential substances must diffuse.

Changes in Lymph Circulation

Lymph flow in normal tissues increases during massage. Drinker (1939) and Drinker and Yoffey (1941) demonstrated on anesthetized dogs that an increased flow of lymph, measured in a cannulated lymph trunk, could be sustained indefinitely for as long as massage of the area drained by the trunk continued. When massage was stopped the lymph flow ceased or was negligible.

In another animal study, Ladd et al. (1952) compared the effects of massage, passive motion, and electrical stimulation on the rate of lymph flow in the foreleg of dogs. All three procedures were found to increase lymph flow greatly over that in a control period, and massage was found to be significantly more effective than either of the other methods. Elkins et al. (1953) similarly found that kneading and stroking massage resulted in a 7- to 9-fold increase in lymph flow rate, whereas heat, infrared, short wave, and microwave diathermy did not increase lymph flow at all. Earlier, Bauer et al. (1933) had shown that proteins injected into joints of dogs were removed by lymphatic vessels and that their elimination was increased as a result of massage and passive motion.

It may be noted that all of the above studies are over a half century old, and it is both interesting and somewhat inexplicable that there has been virtually no recent research in this area. The reader may be assured, however, that the procedures and physiology of these studies are elegant, and that the simplicity of the protocols and the magnitude of the changes recorded procluded the necessity for complex randomizations and sophisticated statistical analyses for their interpretation.

The effect of massage on lymph flow in normal tissues may be explained in terms of Starling's law of capillary fluid dynamics, which states that the net filtration pressure at capillaries is equal to the mean capillary hydrostatic pressure (CHP) plus the interstitial fluid colloid osmotic pressure (ICOP) minus the sum of the blood colloid osmotic pressure (BCOP) and the interstitial fluid hydrostatic pressure (IHP), or:

$$\text{Net Filtration Pressure} = (\text{CHP} + \text{ICOP}) - (\text{BCOP} + \text{IHP})$$

The mechanical pumping action of tissue compression and decompression moves lymph through the lymph vessels and causes repeated emptying and refilling of the lymph capillaries, thereby reducing interstitial fluid hydrostatic pressure. This reduction of IHP promotes an increased net outward movement of fluid from capillaries, resulting in a sustained increase in the rate of lymph formation and removal (Yoffey & Courtice 1956; Starling 1894).

Foldi (1978) suggests two additional mechanisms to explain the results of Drinker's work. Massage opens blood capillaries that were previously closed, increasing the total capillary surface area. Since the normal Starling equilibrium slightly favors a net outward movement of capillary fluid, an increase in the filtrating capillary surface results in an increased rate of lymph formation without disturbance of the equilibrium. Foldi's second suggestion is that the pressure caused by massage temporarily augments venous pressure, which in turn increases the capillary hydrostatic pressure, disturbing the Starling equilibrium in favor of greater filtration and thus increasing the rate of lymph formation. Foldi further explains massage's induction of increased lymph flow when edema is present by suggesting that extralymphatic forces of lymphokinesis (contraction of skeletal muscles) do not utilize the entire transport capacity of the available lymphatic cross-section, but that systematic massage does.

Effects of Massage Therapy in Treatment of Edema

Massage of an edematous patient causes a shift of edema fluid from the tissues to the blood, which would be expected to result in increased urinary volume and increased excretion of substances accumulated in the edematous tissues. These expectations appear to be confirmed by the work of Kurz et al. (1978) using Vodder's (1965) technique of manual lymph drainage (MLD), which was developed for the specific purpose of promoting increased lymph flow from the tissues. Regrettably Kurz et al. (1978) do not provide substantiating data, but they do state that the volume of urine collected after treatment was three to four times that collected before treatment, and report the immediate excretion of up to a liter of urine following one hour of massage to patients with various types of lymphedema. They also report that urine concentrations of various neurohormones (17-hydroxycorticosteroids, adrenaline, serotonin, and 5-HIAA) decreased after MLD, suggesting a dilution effect, and that histamine and noradrenaline concentrations increased, suggesting improved clearance of these substances from edematous tissues. In fact, the increased urine output itself is the most meaningful result reported, and merits further investigation. In a recent animal study, Kriederman et al. (2002) demonstrated the effectiveness of MLD in treating rats with surgically induced unilateral hind-limb edema. They observed a significant reduction in edema over a five day interval.

> *There are numerous reports in the literature of the effectiveness of Manual Lymph Drainage (MLD) in the treatment of edema.*

In contrast, massage of a non-edematous patient would not be expected to result in additional plasma volume or urinary output, since increased lymph formation and removal rates can occur without a net shift of fluid from the interstitial to the intravascular compartments. Nevertheless, some evidence of washout of substances from the interstitial spaces may be expected. Arkko et al. (1983) reported increased serum creatine kinase, lactate dehydrogenase, and serum potassium levels in healthy volunteers following one hour of whole body massage. Changes in plasma volume were ruled out by the finding that total serum protein, hematocrit, hemoglobin, and erythrocyte counts did not change. These results could be interpreted to indicate a flushing out of interstitial fluid by increased lymphatic circulation.

Another interesting result was achieved by Ernst et al. (1987), who report that blood viscosity, hematocrit, and plasma viscosity decreased following a standard 20 minute whole body massage, indicating hemodilution. Two explanations are advanced: that underperfused vessels become filled with cell-free interstitial fluid of low viscosity, which is released to the circulation when the hyperemic response to massage in skin and muscle results in recruiting of these vessels; and/or that simple mechanical compression causes a shift of interstitial fluid into the circulation.

However these findings are finally interpreted, they point to massage's profound effectiveness both in increasing lymph circulation in non-edematous tissues and in bringing about the removal of fluid from edematous tissues.

Clinical Effectiveness

The efficacy of massage therapy in reducing edema in clinical situations is widely recognized. Cyriax (1984a) strongly recommends deep effleurage for relief of edema.

Wakim et al. (1955) showed that simple rhythmic compressions of an edematous limb using a pneumatic cuff was effective treatment for radical mastectomy patients or patients with post-traumatic edema. Similar results were obtained by Valtonen (1967) in patients with post-traumatic edema, diseases of the veins involving deep thrombosis, and idiopathic lymphedema. In a more recent study involving more than 400 patients with edematous limbs, Yamazaki et al. (1988; 1979) confirmed plethysmographically that edema was reduced and blood flow increased by application of a mechanical pneumatic device producing undulatory massage in a proximal direction.

Pflug (1974) reported that intermittent compression therapy and massage greatly reduced postsurgical swelling and pain, and also reduced generalized swelling of the lower limb, rapidly converting pitting to non-pitting edema in cases of locally impaired drainage, cardiac failure, or nephrotic syndrome (Pflug 1975). Therapeutic massage has been found to be particularly effective for reducing digital volume in the treatment of

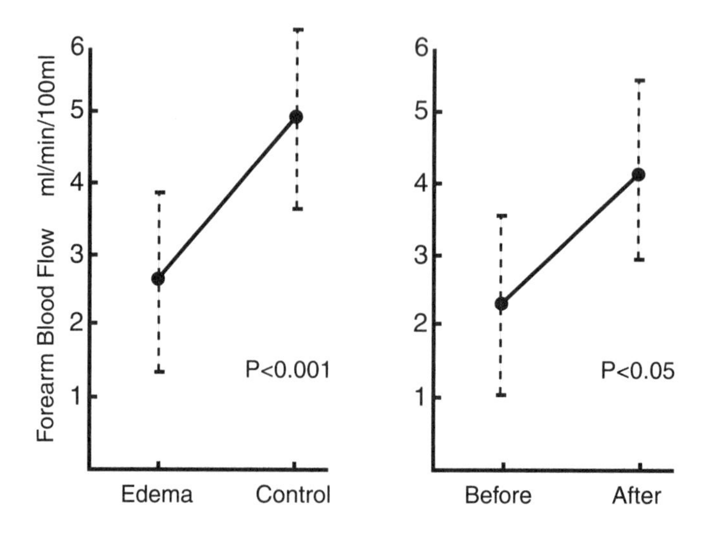

Forearm blood flow of the patients with postmastectomy edema of the arm: edematous and healthy arm before and after massage.

Yamazaki et al. Admittance Plethysmographic Evaluation of Undulatory Massage for the Edematous Limb, *Lymphology, 1979; 12:42 Figure 4.*

hand injuries (Flowers 1988) and cervical and facial edema following surgery and irradiation. (Einfeldt et al. 1986).

Manual lymphatic massage, pneumatic massage with uniform pressure, and pneumatic massage with differentiated pressure were compared by Zanolla et al. (1984) in a study of post-mastectomy edema. A permanent, statistically significant edema reduction was achieved with manual lymphatic massage and with the uniform-pressure pneumatic massage, but not with the differentiated pressure. Gray (1987) describes similar positive results with limb edema in advanced breast cancer patients.

Manual Lymph Drainage (MLD) is a specific technique developed for the purpose of increasing lymph flow to reduce edema. MLD consists of a series of movements of light pressure, often in a circular pattern, that follow the general distribution of lymph vessels draining a body region. The application of light pressure mimics the tissue pressures and other small magnitude forces normally involved in filling of lymph capillaries; the intrinsic smooth muscle contractions and valve components of the larger lymph vessels aid movement of lymph beyond the capillaries without disturbing the vascular circulation or triggering histamine release.

There are numerous reports in the literature of MLD's effectiveness in the treatment of edema. Kaaja & Tiula (1989) have described its successful usage for edema in pregnancy-associated nephrotic syndrome, both pre- and post-partum. Disappearance of edema following treatment was associated with decreased urinary protein loss and increased daily urine output. The effect of one therapy session lasted two to three days, and edema could be controlled by 2 to 4 sessions weekly. MLD followed by compression bandage therapy is reported to result in an average 20% reduction of total arm volume in post-mastectomy patients (Hutzschenreuter et al. 1992, 1991). Williams et al. (2002) found that not only does MLD produce a significant reduction of excess limb volume in the upper arm in women with breast-cancer related lymphedema, but they also noted improvements in emotional function, dyspnea, and sleep disturbance as well. In a study of 43 children with primary lymphedema and 7 with secondary lymphedema treated twice daily over a 4 week period with MLD followed by bandage compression, limb volume was decreased in 47 patients, although no effect was seen in 3 patients with lymphangioma cysticus (Hutzschenreuter & Herpertz 1993).

When diffusion distances increase in edema, blood flow regulation becomes progressively uncoupled from cellular requirements.

Similar positive results have been found by others for treatment of primary lymphedema with MLD or massage (Little & Porch 1998; Morgan et al. 1992; Browse 1986). MLD has also been found to be useful in the management of secondary edema in scleroderma patients (Mainusch 1992). In a case report by Weiss (1998), MLD and compressive bandaging used to treat leg edema secondary to severe distal tibiofibular fracture and related surgeries resulted in a 80.9% decrease at ten weeks after the start of treatment. Howard & Krishnagiri (2001) describe treatment of a patient with multiple trauma in which manual edema mobilization resulted in a 78% reduction in persistent edema in the affected limb.

There are a variety of reports employing combined systems that include massage or MLD as one component. Morgan et al. in 1992 described one such system, known as Complex Physical Therapy for the treatment of the lymphedematous arm, in which two courses of treatment of 4 weeks each separated by one year resulted in a greater than 50% reduction in edema following the first course of treatment and a further reduction of more than 50% of the remainder following the second course. Boris et al. (1997) found that a combined treatment system referred to as Complex Lymphedema Therapy including skin care, compression bandages and stockings, and exercise in addition to MLD reduced arm lymphedema by 62.6% in 56 patients and leg lymphedema by 68.6% in 38 patients. After 36 months the average reductions were 63.8% and 62.7% respectively. Ko et al. (1998) found that a similar system known as Complex Decongestive Physiotherapy, which also combines MLD with skin care, compression bandages, and exercise, produced an average lymphedema reduction of 59.1% in the upper limb and 67.7% in the lower limb. The improvement was maintained at 90% of the initial reduction at follow-up after 9 months. Based on his experience with two thousand lymphedema patients, Lerner (1998) concluded that Complex Decongestive Physiotherapy is superior to surgical procedures and pneumatic pump therapies in the treatment of lymphedema.

Trettin (1993) reported that post-concussion patients receiving MLD report a lessening of head pressure and pain.

MLD has also been reported to be of benefit in applications that do not primarily involve the reduction of edema, although the effects are presumably related to increased clearance of lymph fluid. Trettin (1993) reported that post-concussion patients receiving MLD report a lessening of head pressure and pain. Concentration and alertness are increased, blood pressure decreases, and the tendency to faint or collapse is decreased. Kouri (1992) has found aquatic exercise followed by MLD to have positive effects on symptoms of fibromyalgia, and case reports by Tucker et al. (1998) indicate that 14 MLD treatments of 45 minutes each over a four-week period can result in pain reduction and improved sleep quality for fibromyalgia patients.

Treatment Applications

Local regulation of tissue blood flow is thought to be accomplished by contraction or relaxation of precapillary sphincters in response to changes in oxygen concentration (oxygen demand theory) or in metabolite concentrations in the immediate vicinity of their smooth muscle cells (vasodilator theory).

Under normal circumstances, the distance between capillaries and the tissue cells they supply is relatively small and diffusion can occur rapidly across it; this mechanism assures both an adequate supply of oxygen and nutrients and removal of wastes. However, when extravascular fluid increases, so does the capillary-to-cell distance, and diffusion time increases as the square of the distance. When diffusion distances increase in edema, blood flow regulation becomes progressively uncoupled from cellular requirements. As the metabolic circulation (Ladd et al. 1952) slows, the cellular metabolism may become so impaired that atrophy or death of the cell may occur. Vascular disturbances further aggravate the situation.

Another significant aspect of increased lymphatic circulation, suggested by Pemberton (1950), is that increased flow of lymph can hasten the removal of metabolic products of dysfunction, including the chemical mediators of inflammation, inflammatory exudate, extravasated blood, and the detritus and debris produced by trauma. All of these can be expected to contribute to increased fibrosis if not expediently removed, and there are studies which indicate that when massage is given less fibrosis results (Askew et al. 1983; Bodian 1969).

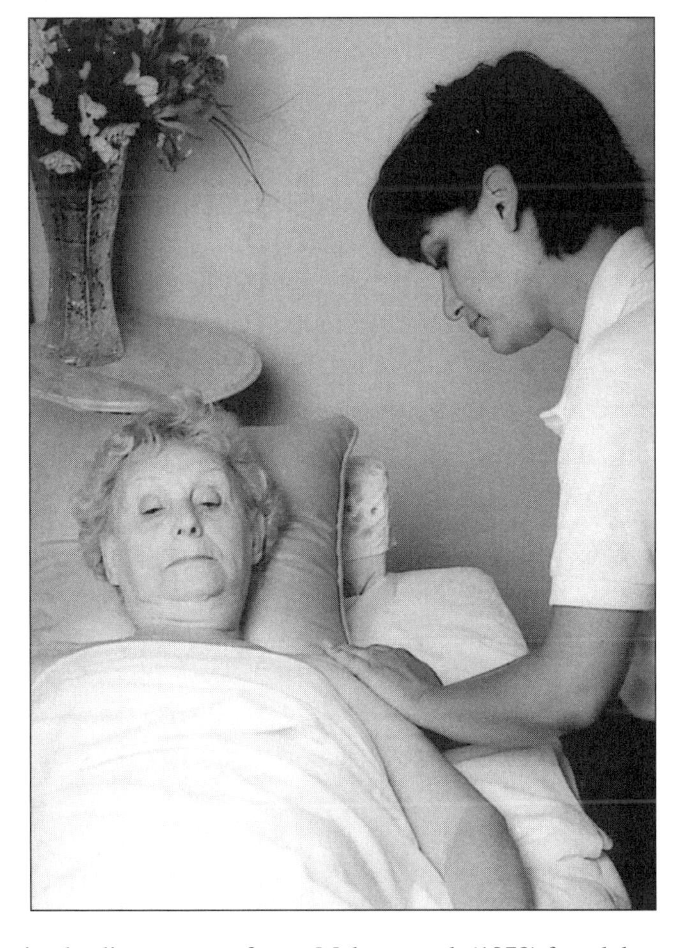

Perfusion also improves as tissue fluid pressure is relieved (Wakim 1976; Scull 1945), and improved drainage restores normal interstitial fluid osmotic pressure (Wakim et al. 1955). This effect may be more important to the healing process than any direct mechanical effect on blood flow.

Clearly, improving lymph circulation and reducing edema are often of considerable therapeutic importance, ultimately allowing healing to occur faster. Melrose et al. (1979) found that intermittent compression therapy increased both the rate and quality of healing when applied to surgical incisions following stripping of varicose veins.

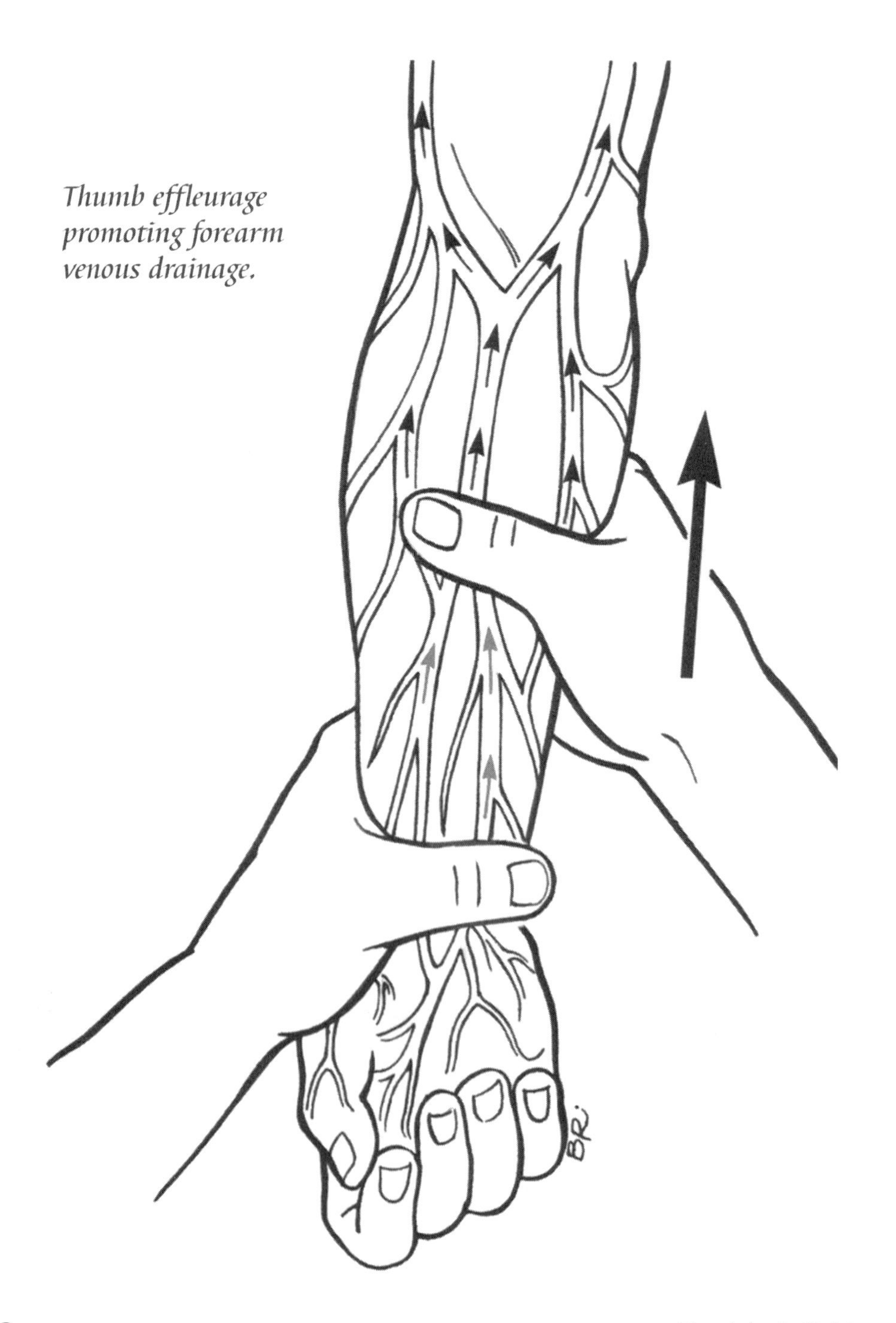

Thumb effleurage promoting forearm venous drainage.

Changes in Blood Circulation

One of the most fundamental and important characteristics of the circulation is the ability of each tissue to adjust its own local blood flow in proportion to its metabolic needs. On purely theoretical grounds, we would expect any changes in local blood flow resulting from massage to be minimal and of short duration in healthy tissue. Provided that mean arterial blood pressure is normal and the arterial circulation unimpaired, local regulation should assure adequate blood flow to supply tissue requirements at any given point in time, and any induced increase in blood flow will be rapidly compensated for by closing of precapillary sphincters.

However, based largely upon the observation of dilation of superficial blood vessels and increases in skin blood flow (Wilkins et al. 1950; Scull 1945), it is commonly believed that massage can increase local blood flow even in normal tissues. Various attempts have been made to verify this effect of massage, with diverse results (Valtonen et al. 1973; Heipertz 1965, 1963; Wakim et al. 1949; Scull 1945), indicating that what changes do occur in deeper tissues, as predicted from theory, are neither dramatic nor highly consistent in normal individuals. Attempts have been made to explain the local blood flow changes that do occur in terms of three types of effects: direct physical and mechanical effects on the tissue vasculature; circulatory changes mediated by the local release of vasodilator chemicals; and circulatory changes elicited by reflex responses of the autonomic nervous system to tissue stimulation.

- ***Physical and Mechanical Effects***

The findings of several researchers (Hansen & Kristensen 1973; Wolfson 1931) seem to support the idea that local increases in blood flow rate caused by massage are produced through mechanical means. Compression of the tissue empties venous beds, lowering venous pressure and increasing capillary blood flow (an effect which should be quickly counteracted in normal tissues as autoregulation returns blood flow rate to the metabolically determined optimum). Venous return and stroke volume are increased as expected in consequence of the enhanced venous flow (Goats 1994; Wakim 1976). Cessation of massage results in an apparent temporary decrease in blood flow during the period when the vascular beds are refilling. These changes have been confirmed by xenon clearance studies showing increased clearance during effleurage and a subsequent decrease following cessation of massage (Hansen & Kristensen 1973). It is important to note that a substantial part of the literature dealing with the circulatory effects of massage represents studies in which no pathology affecting the circulation is involved. It may be that massage has its most readily demonstrated effects upon a compromised circulatory system, which may explain some of the inconsistency in research findings. Any effects which can be substantiated to occur in normal tissues will be of considerably greater significance where conditions are present which impair the circulation. It is reasonable to extrapolate that massage may produce therapeutically significant increases in blood flow through mechanical effects in some conditions of impaired circulation or venous stasis, as has been demonstrated for massage and pneumatic compression in the prevention of venous thrombosis (Cotton & Roberts 1977; Knight & Dawson 1976; Sabri et al. 1971).

- ***Vasodilator Release***

Local blood flow may also be altered by chemically mediated arteriolar and capillary dilation. Histamine is the best known example of such a vasodilator substance. Localized skin hyperemia and an associated increase in skin temperature are consistently observed in response to massage, presumably resulting from the same local vasodilatation mechanism as in the Lewis triple response.

Although Carrier (1922) reported an increase in local blood flow and stroke volume lasting approximately one hour after deep massage, it has never been demonstrated that such increases in blood flow are the result of chemically mediated vasodilation in subcutaneous tissues. To the contrary, evidence that this effect may not be significant subcutaneously is provided by Linde (1986), who found that massage of subcutaneous insulin injection sites markedly increased absorption rates without significantly elevating the subcutaneous blood flow. An immediate marked rise seen in femoral venous blood insulin levels also made it seem unlikely that enhanced lymphatic drainage was the mechanism causing increased absorption. Alternative explanations included improved transport within the interstitial space, presumably resulting from increased movement of fluids, and enlargement of the capillary surface area in contact with the insulin solution, which is consistent with histamine release.

On the other hand, massage can enhance the chemically mediated vasodilator effect of other substances, as shown by Severini & Venerando (1967a). They found that deep massage in combination with a hyperemia-producing drug (containing vanellylin amide and butoxethyl nicotinate) resulted in an increase in muscle blood flow not produced by the drug either alone or in combination with superficial massage. Thus, although massage induced increases in blood flow mediated by the release of histamine or similar vasodilator substances may occur in deeper tissues just as it does in skin, the intensity and duration of this effect in normal subjects is certainly not great, and if it does occur is often not detected.

- ***Reflex Responses in the Autonomic Nervous System***

Changes in blood flow may also be induced by means of autonomic vascular reflexes, in which stimulation of cutaneous or deep-tissue receptors triggers changes in venous or arteriolar tone via the sympathetic efferents, as was suggested by the work of Leroy (1941). Such a mechanism is strongly suggested by distant increases in blood flow and skin temperature of the hands and feet as a result of connective tissue massage (CTM) (Ebner, 1975). Further evidence is provided by several others (Goats & Keir 1991; Gifford & Gifford 1988; Severini & Venerando 1967b; Cuthbertson 1933), whose studies of changes in distant circulation as a result of CTM strongly support the view that massage is capable of exerting reflex effects on tissue blood flow. It follows that similar reflex mechanisms may exist that will induce vascular changes in or near the massage site. On the other hand, Wakim et al. (1955; 1949) obtained similar responses in patients with flaccid limb paralysis, indicating that the effect is not entirely dependent upon spinal reflexes.

Changes in Other Circulatory Parameters

As early as 1899, changes in circulatory parameters were reported to be associated with massage. Edgecombe & Bain (1899) found that petrissage resulted in an initial increase and subsequent decrease in arterial pressure, and an increase in venous pressure. It is unlikely that measurable changes in arterial pressures can be ascribed to mechanical effects for sound physiological reasons. However, reflex effects on the heart and vascular tone may be postulated as causes of changes in systemic circulatory parameters. That such reflex effects do occur is suggested by studies showing that both conventional massage (Barr & Taslitz 1970) and CTM (McKechnie et al. 1983; Kisner & Taslitz 1968) produce changes – usually increases – in blood pressure and heart rate. These are associated with changes indicating increased sympathetic activity, and are therefore considered to be mediated by autonomic nervous system reflexes.

Slow stroking massage has been studied in the context of circulatory parameters by several researchers (Fakouri & Jones 1987; Ashton 1984; Longworth 1982) and has generally been reported to reduce heart rate and blood pressure. Longworth (1982), for example, studied the effect of slow-stroke back massage (60 strokes per minute, two inches on either side of the spinous processes) in 32 normal, healthy female volunteers. Massage lasted six minutes and was preceded and followed by 10-minute quiet rest periods. The measures of effect included an anxiety inventory, heart rate, blood pressure, muscle tension (EMG), galvanic skin response, and skin temperature. Systolic blood pressure decreased significantly during the initial rest period, increased by a small but significant amount during the first three minutes of massage, then decreased again and remained at the level achieved during the initial rest period. Heart rate also decreased significantly during the initial rest period, but increased again during the second three minutes of massage, and had returned to the initial level by the end of the

TABLE 1

MEANS OF PHYSIOLOGIAL INDICATORS

	Day 1			Day 2			Day 3		
	Before Massage	Immediately After	Ten Minutes After	Before Massage	Immediately After	Ten Minutes After	Before Massage	Immediately After	Ten Minutes After
Heart Rate	80.44	76.66	76.86	82.11	77.35	78.11	79.44	74.88	74.77
Skin Temperature	91.69	92.77	93.11	92.55	93.36	93.36	92.08	92.88	93.14
Systolic Blood Pressure	132.44	121.33	-	122.50	115.00	-	127.00	119.44	-
Diastolic Blood Pressure	71.55	66.00	-	85.22	83.55	-	68.00	64.00	-

Effects of Slow Stroking Back Massage on Nursing Home Residents
(Average Age: 73.7)

Fakouri & Jones. Relaxation Rx: Slow Stroke Back Rub,
Journal of Gerontological Nursing, 1987; 13:33

final rest period. The fact that heart rate and systolic blood pressure measurements mirrored each other during the massage period suggests that no change occurred in cardiac output. The author concludes that slow-stroke back massage may be effective for cardiac and hypertensive patients, as well as those with high somatic or psychoemotional arousal.

Fakouri & Jones (1987) have verified that as little as 3 minutes of slow stroke back massage results in a reduced heart rate, reduced systolic and diastolic blood pressures, and increased skin blood flows, which they attribute to a "relaxation response." These investigators found that the decrease in diastolic pressure did not reach statistical significance until massage had been administered on repeated occasions, suggesting a conditioned reduction in anxiety.

More recently, Delaney et al. (2002) found that myofascial trigger point therapy to the head, neck, and shoulder areas, in addition to decreasing muscle tension, is effective in producing a significant decrease in heart rate, systolic and diastolic blood pressure, as well as an improved emotional state, and concluded that the treatment was effective in increasing cardiac parasympathetic activity.

One intriguing but difficult to interpret report describes the restoration of cardiac rhythm from atrial fibrillation in a single patient (Curtis 1994).

Treatment Applications

Utilization of massage to bring about increases in local blood flow is most likely to be of therapeutic value in circumstances where normal blood flow is impaired. Unfortunately, the literature reviewed included no clinical studies of the effects of stroking or kneading massage on blood flow in patients with impaired circulation.

> *Utilization of massage to bring about increases in local blood flow is most likely to be of therapeutic value in circumstances where normal blood flow is impaired.*

The effects of massage on blood flow can be of considerable benefit in cases of limb paralysis. The extremities are largely dependent upon a combination of metabolic heat production and blood flow demand by muscle tissue to ensure adequate warming of passive tissues with low metabolic demand such as skin and connective tissue. In limbs that have sustained extensive damage to nerve or muscle, this effect will be absent and tissue metabolism and metabolic demand for blood flow will be inadequate to maintain normal tissue temperature. The decrease in temperature will further reduce metabolic rate and lead to deterioration of skin and connective tissue structures. Increases in blood flow and temperature induced by any means may be expected to be beneficial under these circumstances. Wakim et al. (1949) found that deep stroking and kneading massage consistently produced increased circulation in limbs affected by flaccid paralysis. Huddleston et al. (1952), using a vasopneumatic device that produces rhythmical compression and decompression, brought about improvement of the discolored, cold, and clammy condition of limbs paralyzed by poliomyelitis.

Another benefit of massage, pointed out by Mennell (1945), is that sustained muscular contraction impairs venous flow – relaxation of the musculature is a first and essential step in improving the blood circulation. Thus massage can indirectly improve blood flow to muscle tissue made ischemic by spasm.

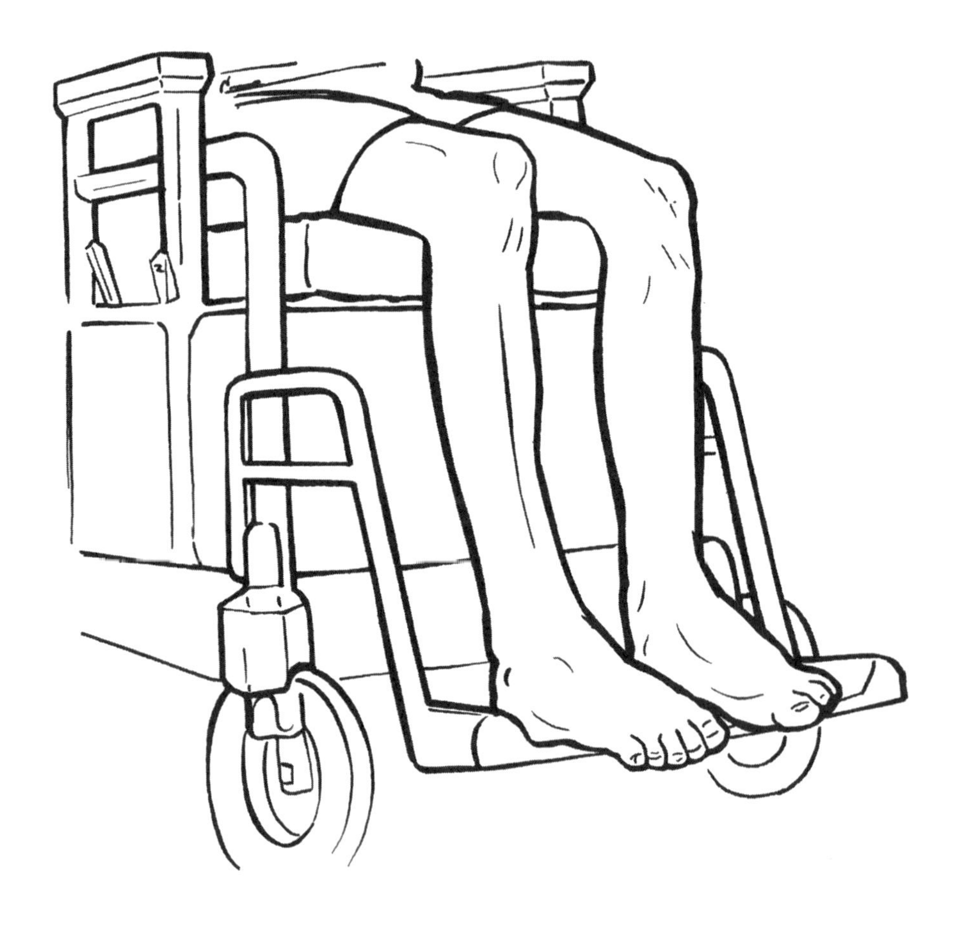

Conditions that Benefit from Massage Therapy's Effects on Blood and Lymph Circulation

By enhancing blood and lymph circulation and decreasing edema, massage hastens the removal of inflammatory by-products and improves the delivery of oxygen and nutrients to the cells. It should be noted that in cases where increasing the circulation by massage may be contraindicated locally, enhancing circulation and drainage proximally (and sometimes distally) can be appropriate and effective.

Pre- and perinatal massage can be of value in reducing edema, decreasing the tendency for development of varicose veins, and generally promoting improved blood and lymph circulation, particularly in the lower extremities.

The circulatory effects of massage are also of great value in the treatment of patients with sinusitis, arteriosclerosis (under stable conditions), and in the prevention of decubitis ulcers. MLD in particular may be indicated for primary and secondary lymphedemas.

Massage therapy may be indicated in conditions involving an acute inflammatory history such as post-operative and post-traumatic edemas (e.g. following mastectomy, fracture, dislocation), in inflammatory conditions in a post-acute stage (e.g. bursitis, whiplash), and in various low-grade inflammatory conditions (e.g. myositis, tendinitis, fibrositis). Examples of other conditions for which massage can be considered an important treatment modality because of enhanced circulation effects include:

- ***carpal tunnel syndrome***
- ***gout***
- ***rheumatoid arthritis and other inflammatory arthritides***
- ***osteoarthritis***
- ***nerve injuries and compression syndromes***
- ***muscular dystrophies***
- ***varicose veins***
- ***Raynaud's Disease***
- ***headaches***
- ***diabetes***
- ***hypertension and congestive heart failure***
- ***contusions***
- ***muscle strain***
- ***ligamentous sprain***

Swedish Massage Technique

Petrissage

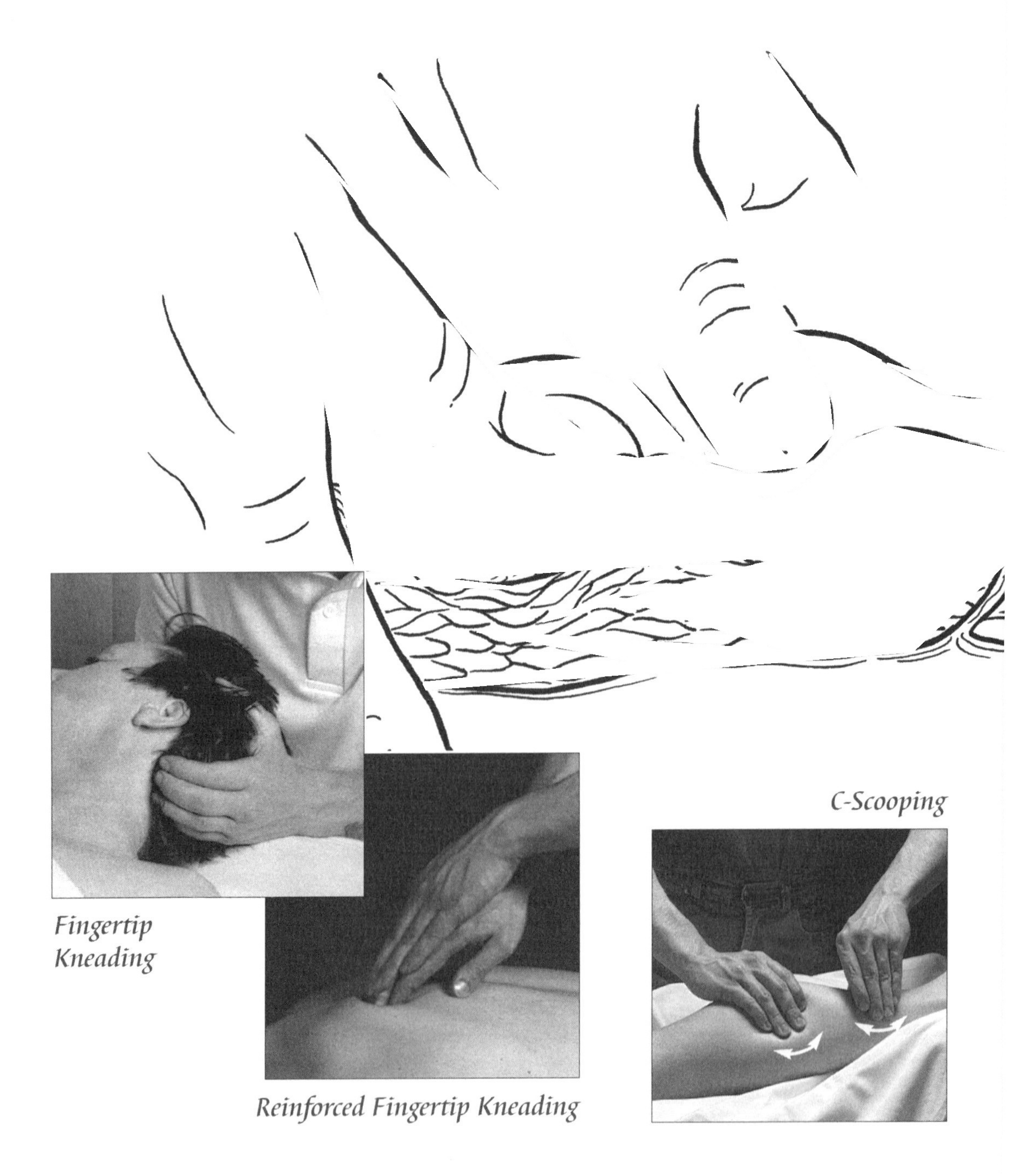

Fingertip Kneading

Reinforced Fingertip Kneading

C-Scooping

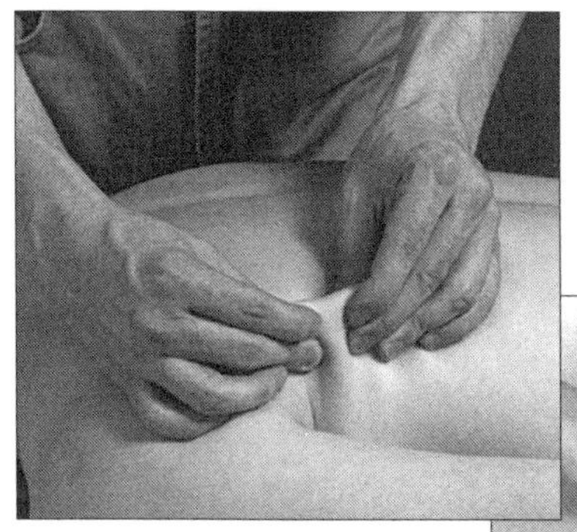

Skin Rolling

Muscle Squeezing

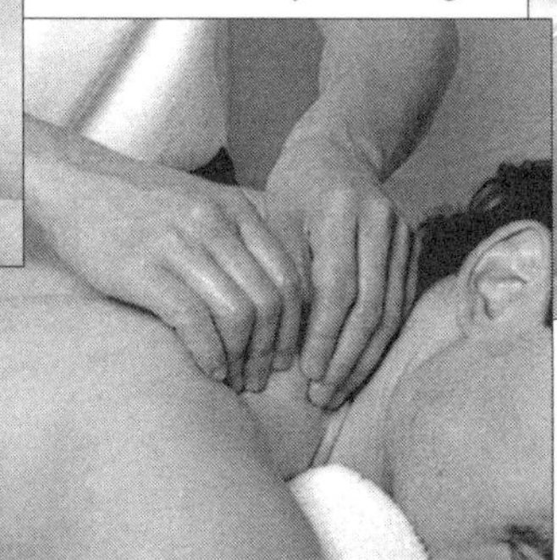

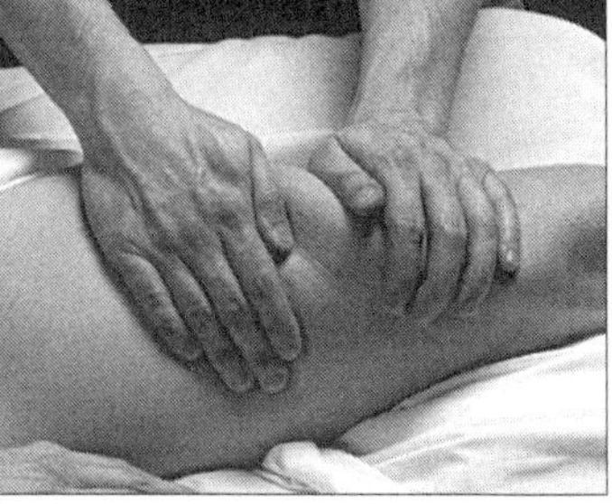

Wringing

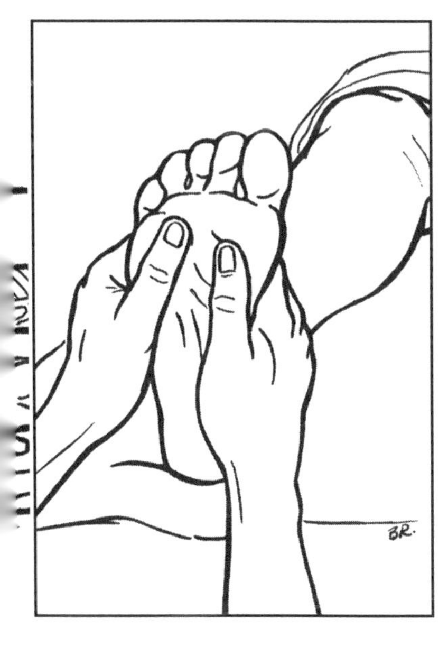

Palmar Kneading

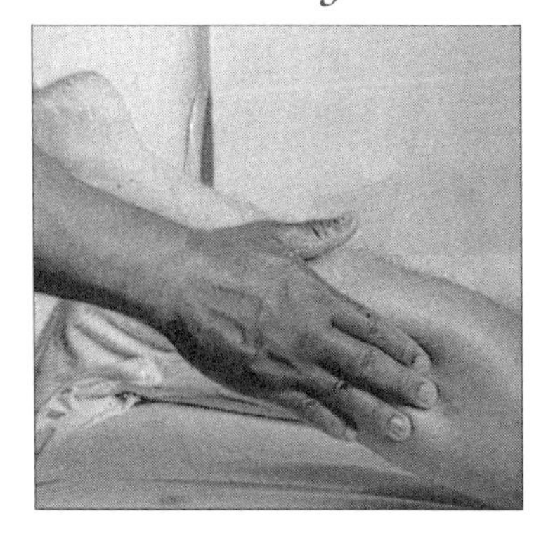

Petrissage LOOSENS/STRETCHES FIBERS

Customary Uses

- Core technique for musculoskeletal complaints, injury rehabilitation, and tension headaches
- Reduces muscle tension and pain; increases joint range of motion
- Improves connective tissue extensibility and mobility; loosens adherences
- Reduces musculoskeletal pain during labor
- Aids peristalsis – treatment of general constipation
- Can be soothing or stimulating depending on rate/rhythm, degree of pressure/drag on tissue

Avoid (AV) or Adapt For (AD)

- AV: Most acute presentations
- AV: Thrombosis, thrombophlebitis
- AV: Hemophilia
- AV: Directly on malignancies or severe varicosities
- AD: Osteoporosis
- AD: Flaccidity, substantial atrophy
- AD: Active trigger point, acute spasm, spasticity
- AD: Anticoagulant, anti-inflammatory, muscle relaxant use

3 Skeletal Muscle

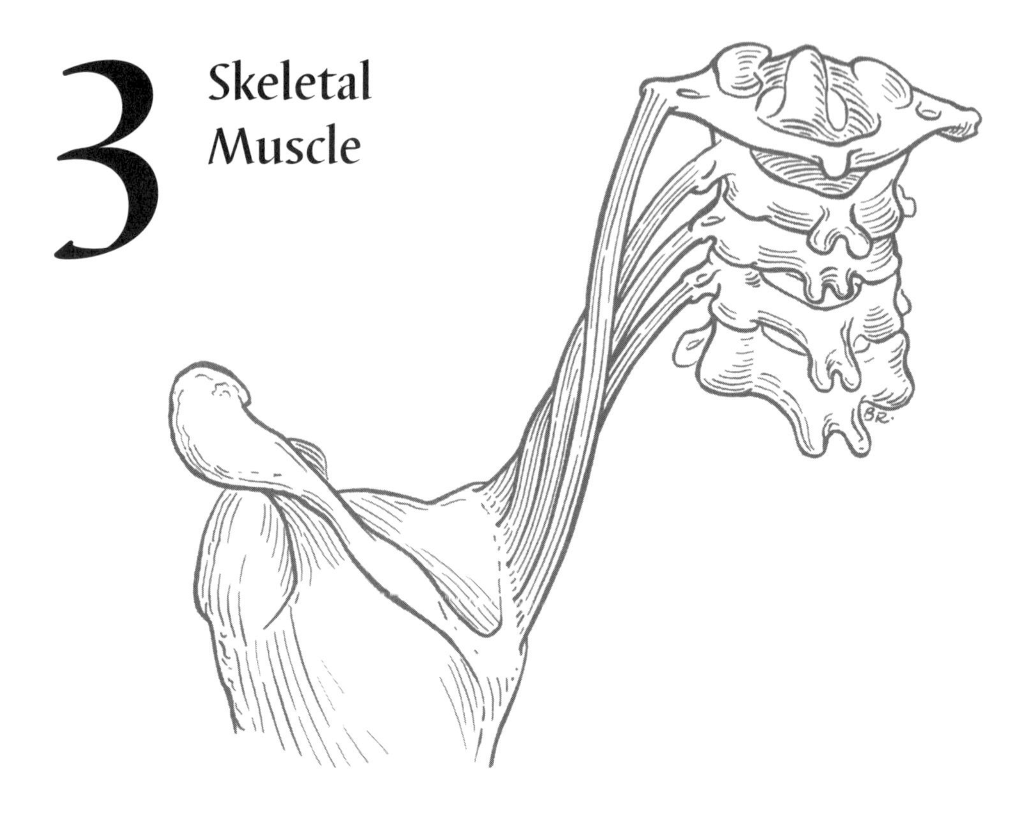

The beneficial effects of massage therapy on skeletal muscle, whether normal or affected by pathology, are generally understood to be:

- muscle relaxation
- relief of muscle spasms/cramps
- treatment of myofascial pain
- prevention or treatment of delayed onset muscle soreness
- improved athletic performance (when massage precedes activity) and enhanced recovery (when applied following training)
- rehabilitation following muscle injury
- treatment of immobilized, paralyzed, and denervated muscles

Muscle Relaxation

That massage induces muscle relaxation is so widely accepted that even a somewhat negative discourse on massage and exercise by Corbett (1972) states: "Massage ... is indeed effective in reducing muscle tension and is often used ... to promote muscle relaxation." Interestingly, the subjective experience of muscle relaxation has been shown by Matheson et al. (1976) not to correlate well with results obtained by EMG monitoring of muscle tension. Objective measurements of muscle relaxation have, however, verified that massage does in fact produce this response.

Nordschow and Bierman (1962) studied the effect of Swedish massage on muscle relaxation in normal subjects as measured by trunk flexion, and found a statistically significant improvement following massage and massage plus rest, but not after rest alone. Twenty years later, Longworth (1982) found electromyographic evidence of muscle relaxation following slow stroke back massage. In this study (described in Chapter 2), the EMG showed a steady decline in muscle activity during the treatment, though it did not become statistically significant until the end of the final rest period.

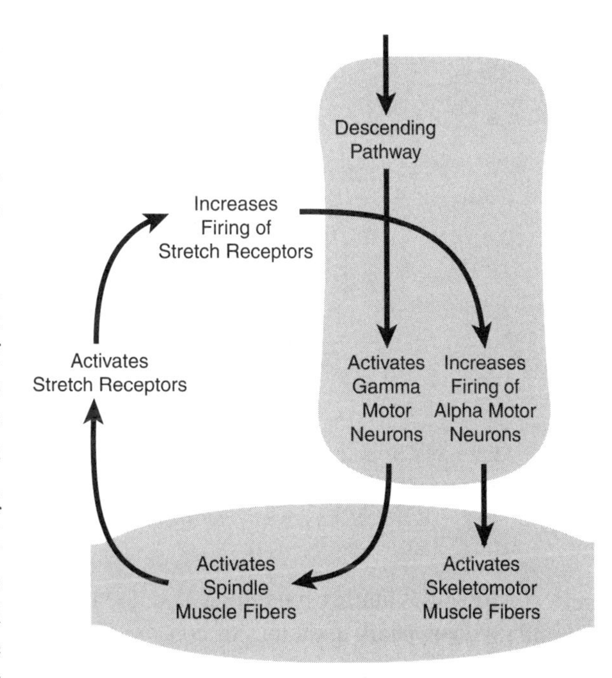

Although, and perhaps because, muscle relaxation is the least disputed of the effects of massage, very little systematic research has been done on the physiological mechanisms that underlie the results. Clearly, since contractile activity of skeletal muscle is entirely controlled by the nervous system, it cannot be altered except by means that influence motor neuron activity – meaning that massage does not affect muscle tone directly. It should also be noted that attempting to separate muscle relaxation from the psychological effects of massage (e.g., anxiety reduction) is probably meaningless. Muscle tone is directed by higher brain centers, and consistently

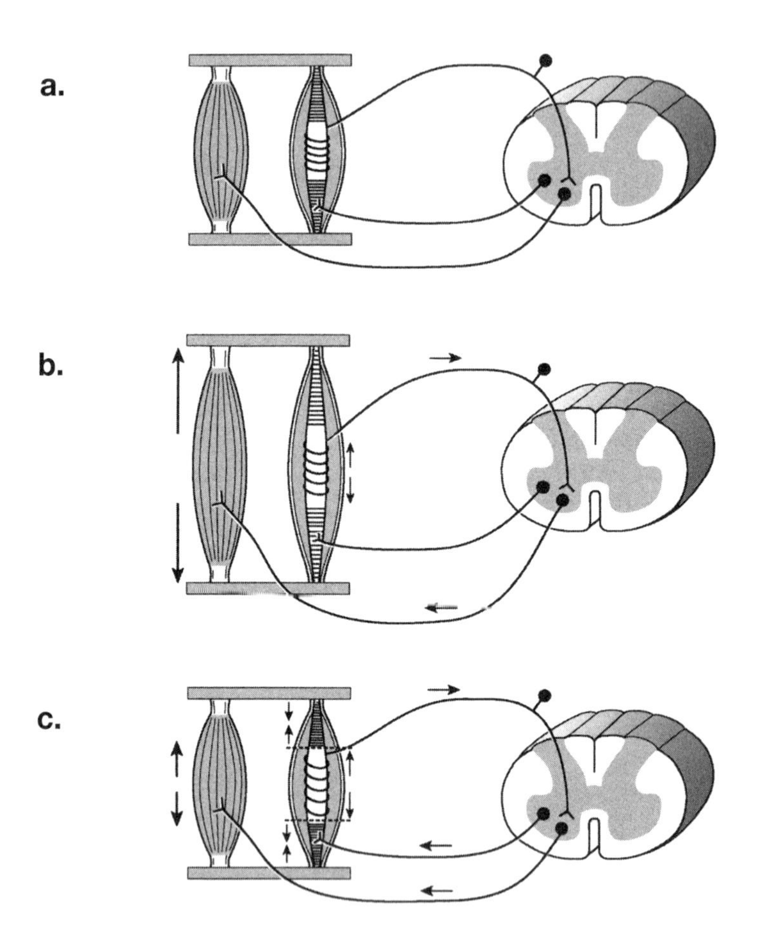

Stretch of a muscle results in sensory afferent firing that produces reflex contraction of the muscle (b, c). When gamma activity is high, the spindle afferents are more sensitive, and a tension-contraction cycle can become established.

reflects the individual's psychological state, as evidenced by the fact that muscle tone essentially disappears upon loss of consciousness.

Resting muscle tone is normally established and maintained via the facilitating effect of muscle spindle activity on the alpha motor neurons. Muscle spindle activity is in turn determined by the rate of firing of the gamma efferent fibers, which are under the direct control of the extrapyramidal system, the reticulospinal tracts in particular. These tracts originate in the nuclei of the brainstem reticular formation, whose level of activity is directly related to the person's psychoemotional state. In deciding to receive massage, an individual makes a voluntary decision to permit passive limb movements and the stretching of muscles by external forces. This necessitates higher brain center inhibition of gamma motor neuron firing so that spindle responses will not cause resistance to muscle elongation by the therapist. The neurophysiology of the relaxation response to massage involves a continuous resetting of resting muscle tone by the reticular formation, until muscle kneading and passive limb movements do not elicit tonic reflex reactions.

Pleasant sensations elicited by massage, together with the psychological effects of being touched in a caring way, must also be expected to impact upon emotional status such that the individual's "readiness for action," manifested as increased resting muscle tone, is reduced.

Establishment of a given level of muscle tone involves more than the facilitating effect of muscle spindle activity. Alpha motor neurons participate in numerous complex reflex arcs involving a wide variety of sensory afferent input, some inhibitory and some excitatory in nature. These stimuli influence alpha motor neuron activity levels, determining whether or not the motor units they control are contributing to muscle tone at any given moment. Whenever a change occurs in sensory transmission into a spinal cord segment, an increase or decrease in motor activity within that segment will follow unless rapid compensatory adjustments are made.

Massage causes a massive increase in sensory input to the spinal cord, so widespread readjustments in these integrated reflex pathways can be expected. It seems reasonable that such a perturbation would spontaneously result in renormalization of imbalances of tonic activity between individual muscles and muscle groups. Thus, where elevated tone has developed in a specific muscle relative to other muscles, because of influences like a sustained posture or emotional state, and has persisted beyond its original cause, the effectiveness of massage may be due in part to increased sensory stimulation.

The results of studies by Goldberg et al. (1994,1992), Sullivan et al. (1991), and Morelli et al. (1990) of the effects of massage on the amplitude of the H-reflex, a monosynaptic reflex elicited by electrically stimulating a nerve, indicate that massage not only reduces the level of motor neuron excitability, but the effect is specific to the muscle group being massaged. The observed inhibitory effect is pressure sensitive, with deep massage bringing about a greater inhibitory response than light massage. Although the decrease in reflex amplitude was also found to occur in subjects with spinal cord injury, there was unfortunately no long-term carryover effect.

Chronic Tension Headaches

Tension headache is an example of a painful condition involving sustained muscle contraction. The headache is thought to be maintained by a pain-tension cycle that must be interrupted in order to bring relief. Chronic tension headaches are difficult to interrupt, and are easily reinitiated because each of the pain and muscle contraction sides of the pain-tension cycle is easily activated.

Massage therapy is widely used in the successful treatment of chronic tension headache, as it combines the effects of relaxing muscle, reducing pain, and resolving hyperirritable foci (trigger points) within muscle. Increased lymph drainage can also be expected, as research cited in the preceding chapter demonstrates, and normalization of blood circulation will tend to occur to the extent that sustained muscle contraction may have compromised blood flow. Improvements in either or both circulatory components will serve to remove metabolites from involved cranial and cervical musculature and fascia. Quinn et al. (2002) conducted a study of chronic tension headache sufferers who had experienced two or three headaches per week for at least six months. Following four weeks of baseline headache measures, subjects received a subsequent four weeks of twice weekly 30-minute massage therapy treatments directed toward neck and shoulder muscles. Compared with baseline values, headache frequency was significantly reduced within the first week of the massage protocol and continued to decrease for the remainder of the study, although headache intensity was unaffected. The authors concluded that the muscle-specific technique used in this study has the potential to be a functional, nonpharmacological intervention for reducing the incidence of chronic tension headache. Puusjarvi et al. (1990) have described another study in which 21 patients were treated for chronic tension headache using trigger point release therapy, deep tissue massage (kneading and stroking), and transverse massage of neck and thenar muscles. Ten massage therapy treatments over two and a half weeks resulted in improved ROM in all directions and a significant pain reduction; the increased number of days without pain was sustained over a six month follow-up period.

> *Massage therapy is widely used in the successful treatment of chronic tension headache, as it combines the effects of relaxing muscle, reducing pain, and resolving hyperirritable foci (trigger points) within muscle.*

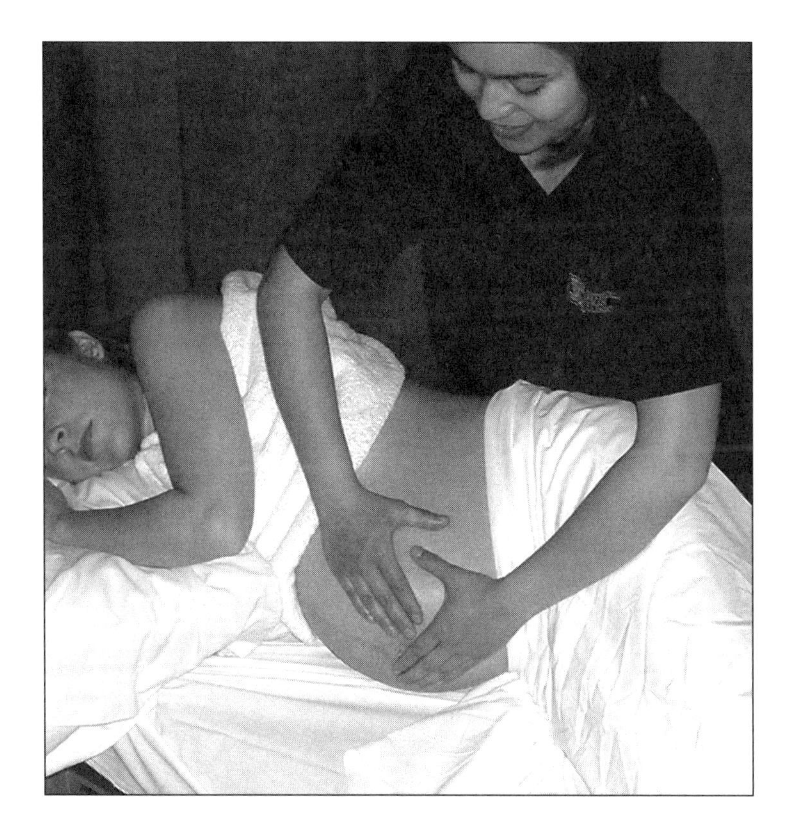

Pregnancy Related Musculoskeletal Pain

It is estimated that 48-56% of expectant mothers have back pain. Approximately 50% is experienced in the sacroiliac area and 25% in each of the upper and lower back regions (Osborne-Sheets 1998). Many pregnant women also develop pain in their feet, legs, hips, and arms. Much of the musculoskeletal pain experienced during pregnancy is from muscle strain secondary to changes in structural balance and posture. These changes establish pain-tension cycles and irritable foci that benefit from massage therapy treatment, including trigger point therapy.

Relief of Spasms and Cramps

Although, surprisingly, we found no studies dealing specifically with muscle cramps, one is reminded that the immediate intuitive response to developing a cramp is to massage the area. A theoretical rationale for massage efficacy can be formulated on the basis of at least two points. Focused elongation of a contracted muscle's tendon can be expected to elicit inhibitory golgi tendon reflex responses, which should contribute quickly to relieving the spasm. Also, improved circulation within the muscle should be directly beneficial through removing metabolic wastes and interrupting the pain-tension cycle that results from ischemia. Stamford (1986) suggests that massage is helpful once the cramp is relieved because it promotes increased blood flow to the tissue areas that had been compromised by vascular compression during the spasm, although this has yet to be confirmed and remains speculative and controversial.

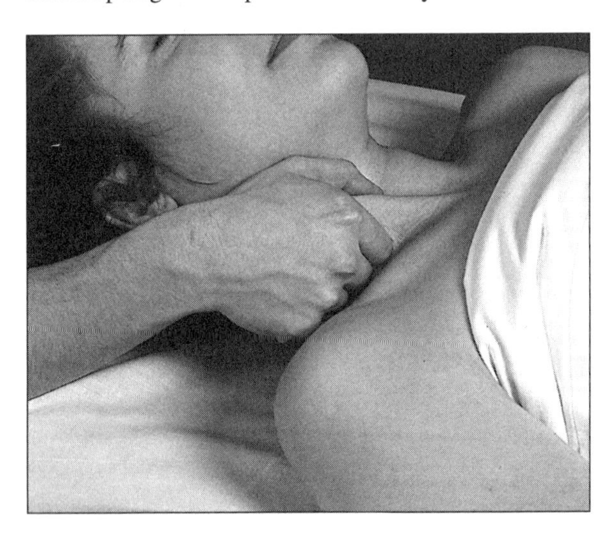

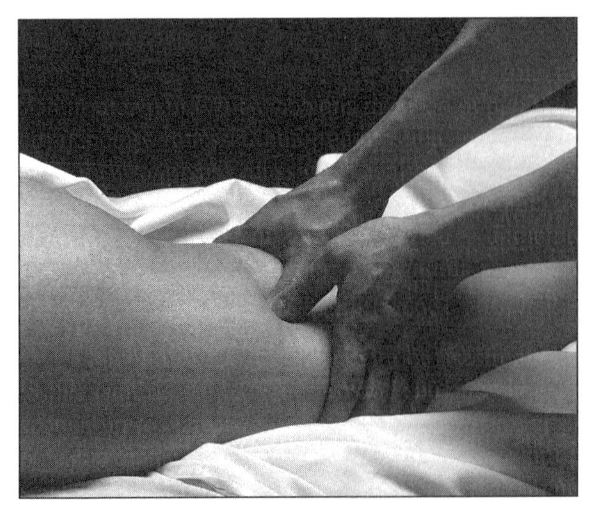

Muscle spasm often involves only part of a muscle. Korr (1975) offers a rationale both for this phenomenon and for its treatment by manipulative techniques. The 'ropiness' that is often observed in painfully tense muscles would seem to represent spasm of selected fascicles, feeling on palpation like tight cords. Given that muscle spindles regulate the contraction of muscle fibers in their immediate vicinity, spasm of selected fascicles would logically result from excessive sensitivity of the muscle spindles controlling them, which would suggest overactivity of the gamma efferents.

Manipulative procedures that stretch overly tonic muscles bring about relaxation mechanisms involving their muscle spindles and golgi tendon organs. Forceful stretching produces two effects:

- Forced stretch against the muscle's spindle-maintained resistance produces a barrage of afferent impulses that signal the CNS to inhibit firing of the gamma motor neurons.
- Tension in the tendon increases, causing intense discharge by the golgi tendon organ. The inhibitory influence of the GTO's afferent input is believed to extend to the gamma as well as the alpha motor neurons, contributing to relaxation of both the intrafusal and extrafusal fibers.

These mechanisms would operate in such muscle-stretching procedures as taking joints through their full range of motion and slowly applying and releasing manual pressure transversely to the long axis of a muscle, as well as in those manipulative techniques in which the patient pushes against opposing force applied by the therapist. Since this latter type of procedure is repeated at incremental muscle lengths, tension develops in the tendons and the spindle is progressively stretched. Both factors contribute to resetting of spindle activity to normal levels.

Myofascial Pain

A plethora of terms, for instance myalgia, myositis, fibrositis, myofibrositis, fibromyositis, fasciitis, myofasciitis, rheumatism, fibrositic nodule, myogelosis, fibropathic syndrome, and myodysneuria, have been used to describe a myofascial pain syndrome that is now most commonly known as the myofascial trigger point. The characteristic lesion is a hyperirritable spot, usually within a taut band of skeletal muscle or in the muscle's fascia, that is painful on compression and gives rise to characteristic referred pain, tenderness, and autonomic phenomena. A trigger point may be induced by trauma or strain, local chilling, poor posture, or fatigue or tension of the muscle. This phenomenon has been thoroughly described by Travell and Simons (1983).

Myofascial trigger points can be effectively treated through the application of focal deep pressure and massage over the trigger point (Travell and Simons 1986, 1983). Although no quantitative studies of this treatment method were located, it has been suggested that the applied pressure stimulates proprioceptive nerve endings, which facilitate enkephalin release and pain modulation. It is also thought that the stretching of musculotendinous structures via tissue kneading initiates reflex muscle relaxation as outlined in the previous section (Swezey 1983).

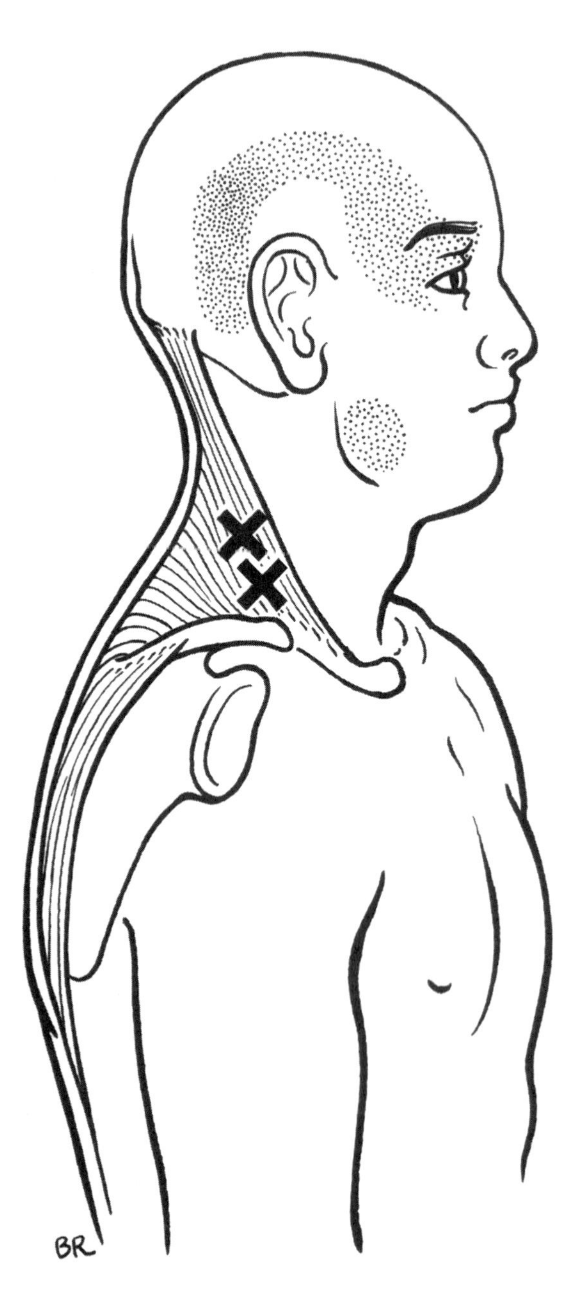

Common headache and jaw pain inducing trapezius trigger points.

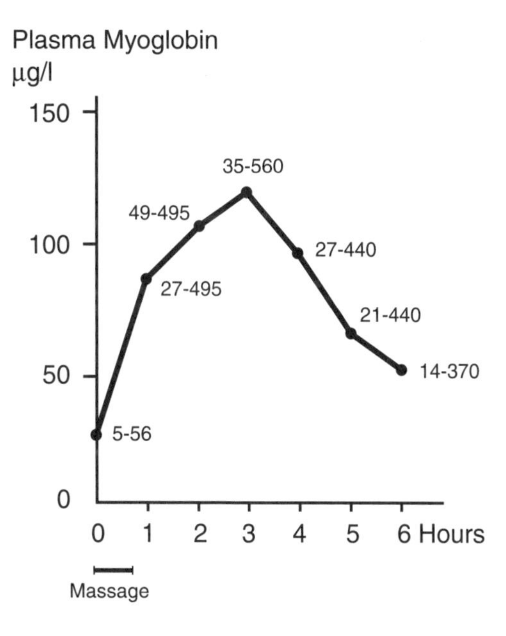

Danneskiold-Samsoe B, Christianson E, Lund B, Anderson RB,
Regional Muscle Tension and Pain (Fibrositis). Effect of Massage on Myoglobin in Plasma.
Scandinavian Journal of Rehabilitation Medicine, 1982; 15:18.

Danneskiold-Samsoe et al. (1982) studied 13 patients with regional muscle tension associated with myofascial trigger points. Plasma myoglobin concentrations were measured throughout a course of therapy consisting of ten massage treatments of 30-45 minutes duration that were evenly distributed over a four week period. A positive correlation was found between degree of muscle tension and increase in plasma myoglobin concentration following massage; massage of non-tender, non-painful muscles did not increase myoglobin concentrations. Both the index of muscle tension and the increases in plasma myoglobin concentration declined after repeated massage treatments. The rise in myoglobin became significant after the first massage treatment, and the effect on index of muscle tension became significant after the fourth. Both effects plateaued after the seventh treatment, and plasma myoglobin concentrations were not different from control following the tenth treatment. The authors concluded that massage is effective in normalizing muscle tension.

A subsequent study (Danneskiold-Samsoe et al. 1986) of 26 patients with myofascial pain produced similar results. In the 21 subjects for whom treatment was successful, massage again produced an increase in plasma myoglobin. After repeated massage treatments muscle tension and pain decreased, paralleled by a decline in the elevated myoglobin levels produced by massage. The authors suggest that the observed post-massage increase in plasma myoglobin indicates that it is leaking from the muscle fibers, and further, that myofascial pain is a disorder of muscle fibers rather than of intramuscular connective tissue.

They refer to a study by Fassbender & Wegner (1973), who examined fibrositic trapezius biopsy material under an electron microscope and found degenerated mitochondria and increased glycogen deposition in the muscle fibers, indicating a state of hypoxia. It may be that hypoxia damages the muscle cell membrane, with a resultant loss of myoglobin. According to this interpretation, the appearance of myoglobin in plasma following massage is a sign of the pathological process. It is not suggested that the myoglobin gives rise to pain, nor that the benefit of massage is related to its removal. The pain is considered to result from tissue ischemia, and massage works by allowing restoration of normal tissue blood supply.

Bale and James (1991) found post-exercise effleurage to be more effective than rest or a conventional warm-down program in reducing muscle soreness.

In the five subjects for whom treatment did not succeed in reducing muscle tension and pain, no increase in myoglobin was seen following massage, suggesting that these patients were suffering from a different muscle problem. If the above interpretation of the role of ischemia in myofascial pain is correct, ischemia was neither the cause nor the result of the muscle tension and pain in these five patients.

Delayed Muscle Soreness and Muscle Strain

Intense muscular discomfort occurring 24-48 hours following exercise, distinctly different from transient acute pain during or immediately following vigorous exercise, has been identified in the literature as 'delayed muscle soreness' (DMS). This condition is most likely to be seen in individuals who have been inactive for extended periods and engage in sporadic physical exercise, in those who attempt new or unusual types of exercise, and in athletes who abruptly increase their training intensity.

Bale and James (1991) found post-exercise effleurage to be more effective than rest or a conventional warm-down program in reducing muscle soreness. Farr et al. (2002) investigated the effect of massage on DMS induced by downhill walking using one leg as a control while treating the other. Subjects showed significantly less pain in the massaged limb at 24 hours. That massage therapy is beneficial in reducing the pain component of DMS has also been repeatedly demonstrated by others (Hilbert et al. 2003; Hemmings et al. 2000; Ernst 1998; Tiidus et al. 1995; Rodenburg et al. 1994; Smith et al. 1994), although not in every case (Ellison et al. 1992).

As of this writing, neither the physiological basis for DMS nor the mechanisms by which massage therapy is of benefit have been clearly demonstrated. Various theories have been proposed to explain the pathophysiology of DMS:

- A sustained pain-tension cycle involving muscle spasm that results from tissue ischemia, possibly involving the agency of pain-inducing substances released in response to the ischemia, and in which the spasm in turn maintains the ischemia. This theory regards DMS as another form of muscle spasm, and the mechanism by which massage is beneficial is presumably as discussed earlier.
- Structural damage to connective tissue, particularly with eccentric contractions, and/or damage to the muscle fibers (torn tissue theory), possibly involving release of creatinine kinase. Exercise-induced injury in normal muscles has been confirmed in both humans and animals, and eccentric contractions have been shown to produce more fiber degeneration than concentric or isometric contractions (St.-Pierre and Gardiner 1987).
- Accumulation of metabolic wastes and/or inflammatory by-products that produce pain by sensitizing A-delta and C fibers.
- Intramuscular edema activating mechanoreceptors responsible for pain.

What these proposed mechanisms have in common is the supposition of accumulation of some substance or another within the tissue space, be it mediators of inflammatory response or some other product of tissue damage, metabolic waste products, or, as in the last theory, simple fluid volume. On the assumption that the soreness and stiffness associated with DMS follow upon some type of accumulation in the tissue, research has naturally focused on the questions of whether and how massage might result in an accelerated clearance of the substance(s) in question (Yackzan et al. 1984).

Unfortunately this issue has been confused by a controversy that has developed based upon negative or inconclusive results involving blood circulation as the key mechanism for achieving tissue clearance, including intimations that there may in fact be no effect, inasmuch as perception of soreness is subjective in nature.

The reasoning that has resulted in most massage mechanism research in this area exclusively examining blood circulation, changes in blood flow, and changes in blood concentration of various substances is faulty on at least two counts:

1. As was discussed in Chapter 2, there is no physiological reason to expect any significant increase in muscle blood flow from massage, *excepting where there are factors present that can be expected to impair normal blood flow*. There is considerable research evidence to support this conclusion (Goats 1994; Wakim 1976; Hansen & Kristensen 1973; Valtonen et al. 1973; Heipertz 1965, 1963; Wakim et al. 1949; Scull 1945).
2. This recent research has consistently ignored the 'other' circulatory system, the lymphatic system, which has long been known to be greatly enhanced by massage (Foldi 1978; Yoffey & Courtice 1956; Elkins et al. 1953; Ladd et al. 1952; Drinker & Yoffey 1941; Drinker 1939), and to provide a more than adequate mechanism for tissue clearance of pain-inducing substances and fluid (Arkko et al. 1983; Kurz et al. 1978; Valtonen 1967; Wakim et al. 1955; Bauer et al. 1933).

The physiological effects of massage that produce relief from both DMS and muscle strain might reasonably be assumed to be related to some combination of reduction of spasm and swelling, removal of exudates and metabolic wastes through increased lymph flow, and restoration of blood circulation to whatever extent it may have been impaired by spasm. Following reports by Krilov et al. (1985) and Paikov (1985) that massage is more effective in reducing DMS when given a few hours after eccentric exercise, yet another explanation has been proposed. Smith et al. (1994) confirmed the previous results and found that decreased soreness ratings were associated with reduced serum creatine kinase levels and a sustained increase in blood neutrophils. Blood neutrophils were increased as compared to pre-exercise levels in both massage and control groups (the increase presumably initiated in response to muscle tissue damage) and decreased linearly in the control group over the next eight hours as would be expected due to emigration of neutrophils into the muscle. The sustained elevation of blood neutrophils in the massage group suggests, however, that the mechanical action of massage interferes with neutrophil emigration into the injured muscle, thereby moderating the severity of the inflammatory response and subsequent soreness.

Athletic Performance and Recovery

It is widely believed among athletes, coaches, and trainers that recovery following training is facilitated by massage. Massage therapy and hydrotherapy are also recommended for eliminating the consequences of overtraining (SPORTS 1986a).

Early direct evidence of enhanced muscle recovery is provided by the work of Graham (1913), who observed that exercised muscles massaged after fatigue sets in regain vigor sooner and are able to do more work than muscles that are not massaged; and further, that massaged muscles are supple and pliant during their recovery period, whereas unmassaged muscles are stiff. Cuthbertson (1933) also showed that a muscle fatigued by work or electrical stimulation can be restored more quickly and thoroughly by massage than by rest of the same duration, and concluded that massage may be useful in enabling a muscle to perform more exercise. More recently, Viitasalo et al. (1995) reported that post-exercise water-jet massage resulted in less performance decline during repeated intensive training sessions. As well, creatine kinase and myoglobin clearance from muscle was increased, although subjective DMS was not significantly different.

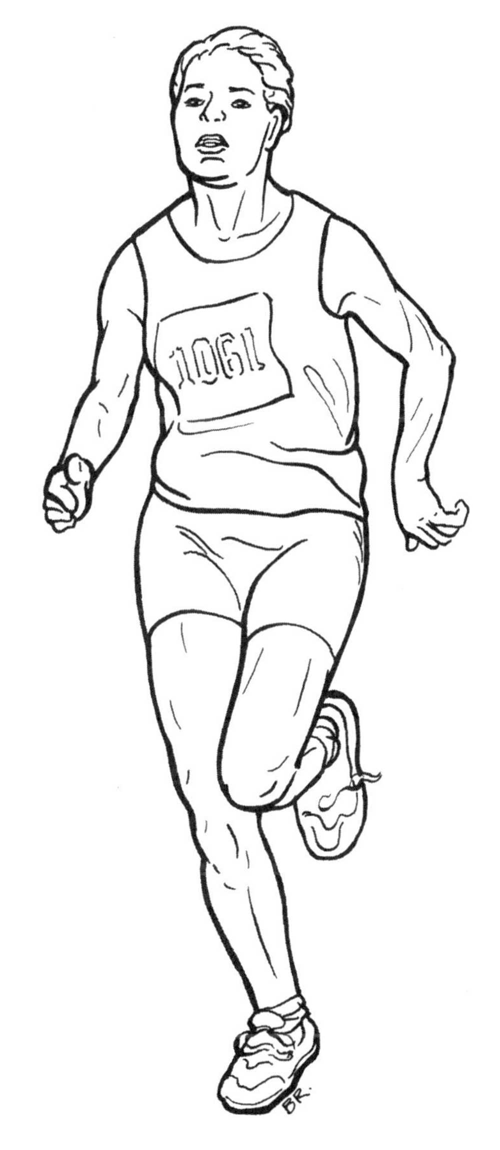

The mechanisms underlying the beneficial effects of massage in athletics are postulated to be enhanced blood and lymph circulation and consequent improved removal of tissue wastes, plus stretching to disrupt adhesions and/or prevent their formation (Newman 1986b). There is ample evidence gathered over nearly a century of research (Zanolla et al. 1984; Yamazaki et al. 1979; Foldi 1978; Kurtz et al. 1978; Valtonen 1967; Vodder 1965; Wakim et al. 1955; Ladd et al. 1952; Drinker & Yoffey 1941; Drinker 1939; Bauer et al. 1933) supporting the contention that lymph circulation and removal of wastes is facilitated by massage (Arkko et al. 1983;

SPORTS 1986b). The effects of massage therapy on adhesions in muscle are discussed in the next chapter.

Pre-exercise massage is often used to reduce the risk of athletic injury. Increased extensibility of soft tissue, including muscle, tendon, fascia, joint capsule, and ligamentous structures, has been described as a direct mechanical effect of massage (Jacobs 1960). A comparative study (Wiktorsson-Moller et al. 1983) showed that massage has a significant beneficial effect on flexibility and is more effective than warm-up exercises. Massage of the hamstring muscle group has also been demonstrated to increase range of motion (Crosman et al. 1984).

A large number of athletes and coaches experience value from massage therapy (Newman 1986a,b) and choose to incorporate it in their programs.

A large number of athletes and coaches experience value from massage therapy (Newman 1986a, b) and choose to incorporate it in their programs. In an article outlining the extent to which Canadian athletes use massage, Newman (1986a) states that more athletes than ever before are receiving massage in conjunction with their training regimes. It is utilized routinely in cycling, and increasingly in track and field, swimming, speedskating, and alpine skiing. Elsewhere, target shooters (Korea) and volleyball players (the Netherlands and Italy) employ massage as a part of their regimens at home and on the road.

The beneficial effects of massage on recovery of muscle tissue following injury (Castex 1891), and on muscle atrophy caused by disuse (St.-Pierre & Gardiner 1987; Chor & Dolkart 1936) or denervation (Wood & Becker 1981; Suskind et al. 1946; Chor et al. 1939) are all, by and large, attributable to prevention or reduction of fibrosis, and are discussed in the upcoming chapter addressing that subject. Massage and passive movement of denervated muscle in particular have been demonstrated to be beneficial in reducing fibrosis during the period required for renervation to occur (Chor et al. 1939). This is an effect of considerable value and importance in treatment following peripheral nerve damage.

An extensive range of musculoskeletal conditions involving various degrees of pain and reduced range of motion are routinely treated by massage therapists, but systematic investigation of these common treatment protocols is rare. One example is a recent study by van den Dolder et al. (2003) in which 29 patients referred to physiotherapy for shoulder pain were randomly assigned to a treatment group that received six soft tissue massage treatments or to a control group that did not. The treatment group showed significant improvements in abduction, flexion, and hand-behind-back range of motion compared to the control group. Massage reduced pain as reported on the Short Form McGill Pain Questionnaire and on the visual analogue scale. The authors conclude that soft tissue massage of the shoulder area structures is effective in improving range of motion, pain, and function in patients with shoulder pain. There is a great need for more such research.

Muscle-Related Conditions that Benefit from Massage Therapy

Massage therapy may be considered the treatment of choice for conditions such as:

- ***muscle spasm***
- ***chronically elevated muscle tone***
- ***tension headache***
- ***myofascial trigger point syndromes***
- ***tight, shortened muscles related to abnormal spinal curvatures (e.g., hyperlordosis, hyperkyphosis, scoliosis), respiratory disorders (e.g., bronchial asthma, emphysema), or postural problems***
- ***muscle-related discomforts of pregnancy***
- ***torticollis***
- ***whiplash***
- ***temporomandibular joint dysfunction***
- ***muscle soreness related to overuse injury incurred during work, sports activities, etc.***
- ***thoracic outlet syndrome (where musculoskeletal elements are causing the problem)***
- ***muscle spasticity of upper motor neuron lesions***
- ***maintenance of muscle tissue during peripheral denervation***
- ***in musculoskeletal injury rehabilitation generally***

Friction

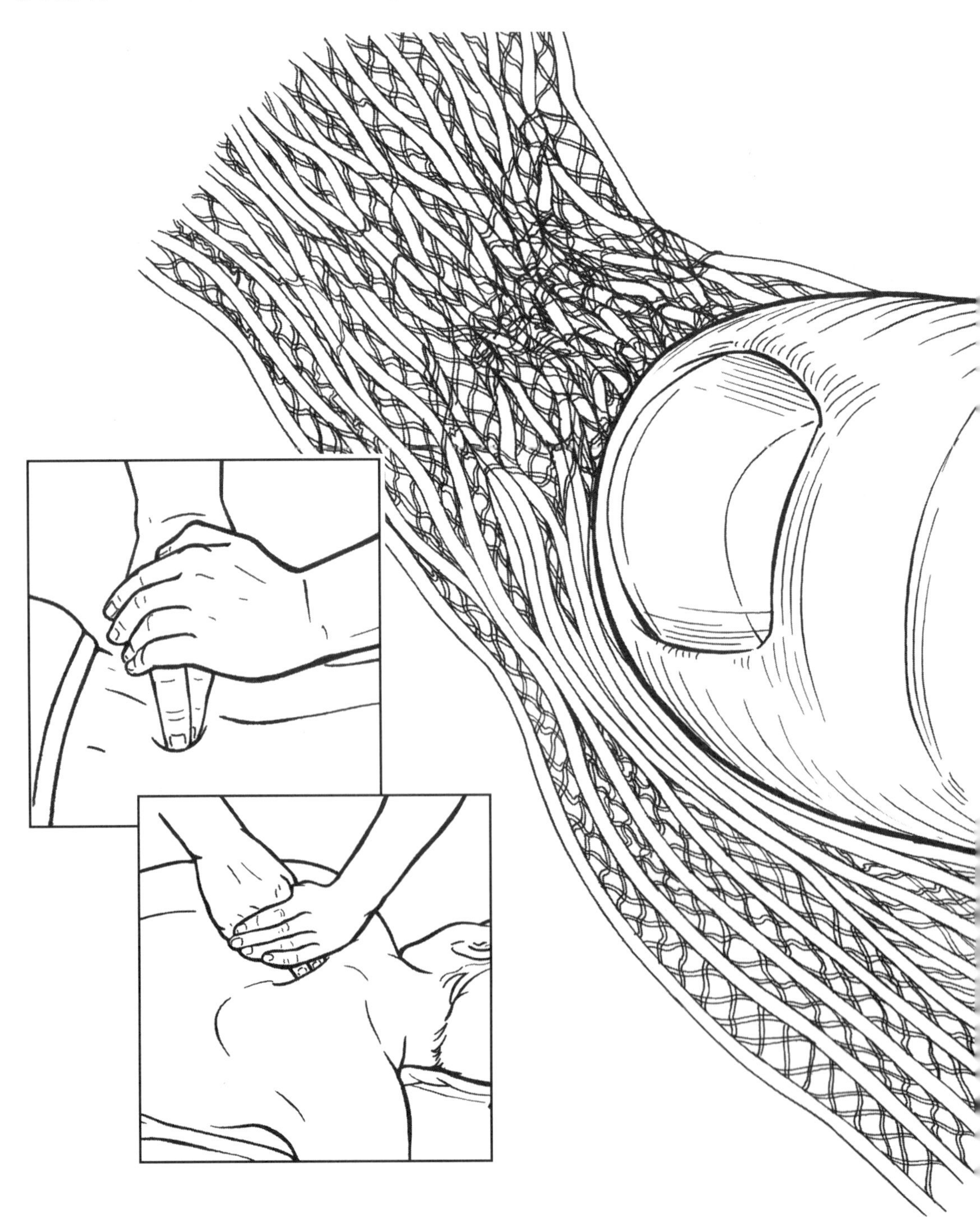

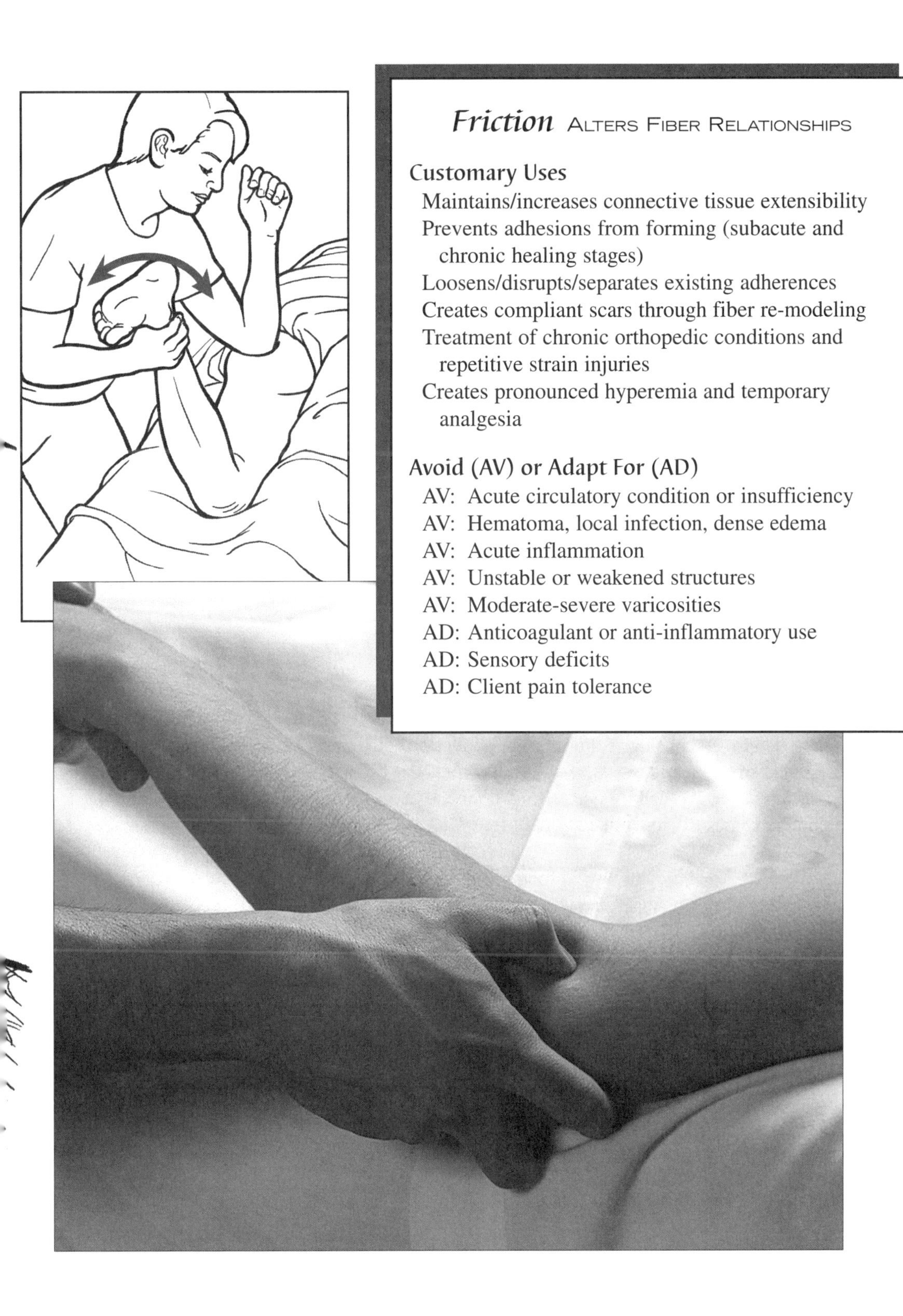

Friction Alters Fiber Relationships

Customary Uses

Maintains/increases connective tissue extensibility
Prevents adhesions from forming (subacute and chronic healing stages)
Loosens/disrupts/separates existing adherences
Creates compliant scars through fiber re-modeling
Treatment of chronic orthopedic conditions and repetitive strain injuries
Creates pronounced hyperemia and temporary analgesia

Avoid (AV) or Adapt For (AD)

AV: Acute circulatory condition or insufficiency
AV: Hematoma, local infection, dense edema
AV: Acute inflammation
AV: Unstable or weakened structures
AV: Moderate-severe varicosities
AD: Anticoagulant or anti-inflammatory use
AD: Sensory deficits
AD: Client pain tolerance

4 Fibrosis and Contracture

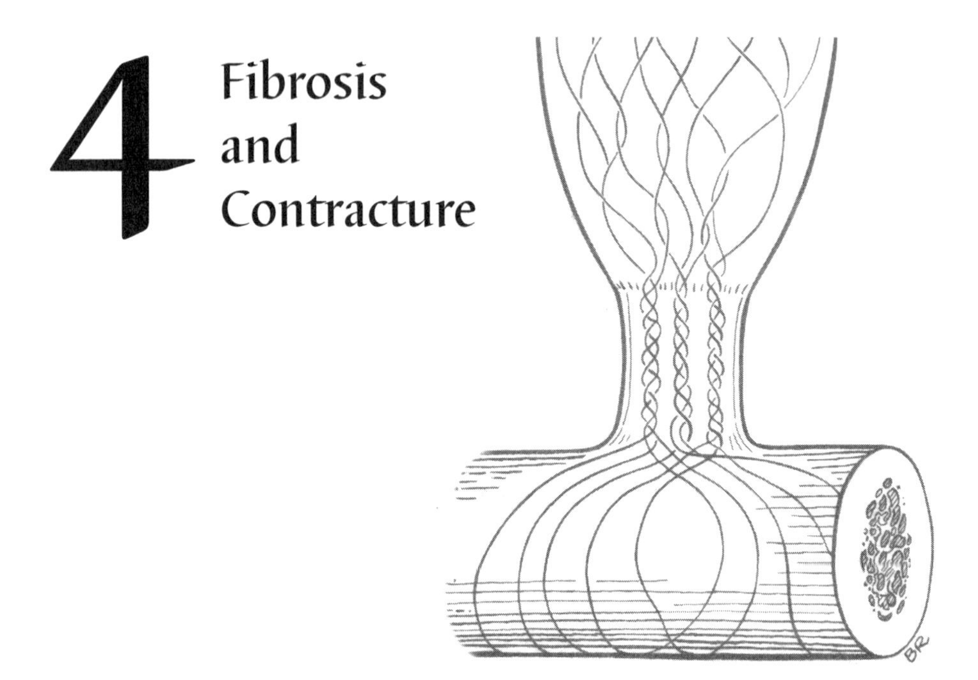

Fibrosis – the formation of abnormal collagenous connective tissue – results from tissue damage, acute or chronic inflammation, infection, sustained or frequently repeated mechanical stresses, and immobilization. Fibrosis is a broad term for various sources of decreased tissue extensibility affecting connective tissue/fascial components, all of which tend to negatively influence pain free range of motion:

- scarring, which is abundant collagen production at repair sites
- an increase in cross-linking among collagen fibers that occurs during immobilization
- formation of fibrous adhesions between structures that are not normally adherent to each other
- contracture (passive shortening of connective tissue elements) that develops with prolonged immobilization or denervation, resulting in loss of elasticity of fascial tissue and adhesion formation
- a consequence of decreased hyaluronic acid production associated with normal aging

Wood and Becker (1981) prescribe massage treatment of muscles subject to fibrosis because of immobilization, injury, or denervation. By using kneading and friction before fibrosis has become extensive, the massage therapist can apply stresses to the tissue that prevent adhesions from establishing and break down early-stage formations. Massage thereby reduces the extent of fibrosis resulting from injury and immobilization, and maintains the elasticity of denervated muscle.

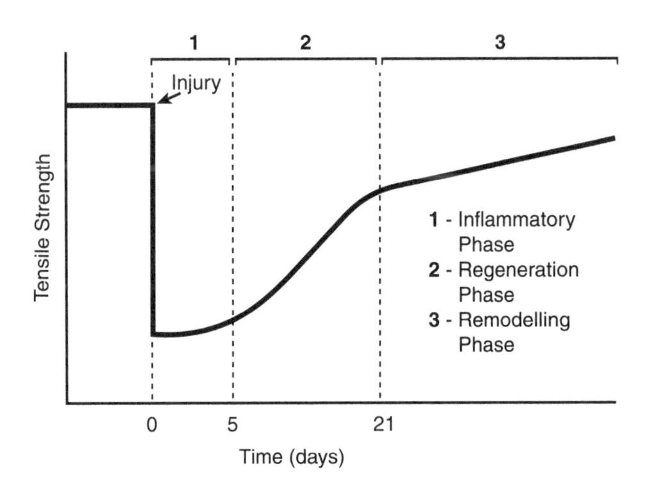

The validity of this treatment concept has been demonstrated in animal studies. Over a century ago, Castex (1891) performed a series of experiments in which animal muscles were subjected to crushing injury; massage was given to one group, while a second was used as a control. When tissue from both groups was examined, it was found that the unmassaged muscles showed hyperplasia and thickening of connective tissue components, whereas the massaged muscle appeared normal. Chor et al. (1939) found that, although atrophy and degeneration of denervated muscle progress despite treatment, massage and passive movement helped to reduce fibrosis during the period required for reinnervation to occur.

The principle techniques employed in the prevention and treatment of fibrosis – used for capsular, ligamentous and tendinous tissues as well as muscle and fascia – are kneading, passive movement (including therapeutic stretch and joint mobilizations), connective tissue massage (CTM), and deep friction massage (Andrade & Clifford 2001).

- *Kneading* brings about a gentle stretching of muscle tissue and produces movement of individual muscles and their enveloping fascia with respect to adjacent structures.

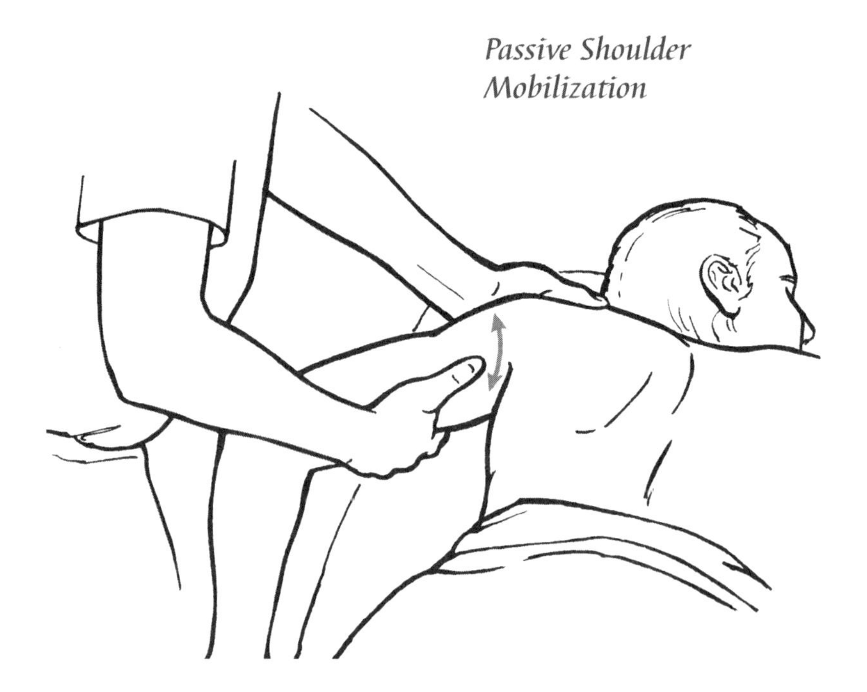

Passive Shoulder Mobilization

- *Passive movements* are used to break adhesions, to stretch joint capsules, muscles and tendons, to maintain range of motion in joints whose muscles are damaged or paralyzed, and to maintain or restore movement after surgery or injury (Cyriax, 1984b).
- *CTM* is a deep fascial mobilizing technique used to relieve pain and overcome movement restrictions from post-traumatic, post-surgical, or postural contractures. The effects attributable to deep friction massage, which are discussed in more detail below, are stretching of contractures, specific mobilization of connective tissue structures, and stimulation of reflex analgesia.
- *Deep friction massage* deliberately causes targeted tissue damage, with concomitant hyperemia and mild tissue inflammation. During the subsequent healing phase, collagen fibrils are encouraged to realign in patterns better adapted to function by careful positioning and exercise.
- *Therapeutic exercise* is used to preserve or increase muscle endurance and strength while preventing adhesions and improving range of motion.

Deep Friction Massage

Deep friction massage has many advocates. In his extensive review of the subject, Chamberlain (1982) discusses both the rationale for maintaining mobility within connective tissue during healing and the case for using friction massage. Corbett (1972) believes it to be the most useful form of massage, effective in chronic supraspinatous tendinitis, some forms of tenosynovitis, ligamentous sprains at the knee and ankle, and medial or lateral epicondylitis. Swezey (1983) describes deep friction massage as a specific therapy for tendinitis to restore pain free motion of tendons and at tendinous attachments, with epicondylitis and biceps tendinitis as the most common indications. Although Cyriax (1960) identifies bursitis as a contraindication for deep friction techniques, Hammer (1993) recommends the use of transverse friction massage in the treatment of chronic bursitis of the hip and shoulder.

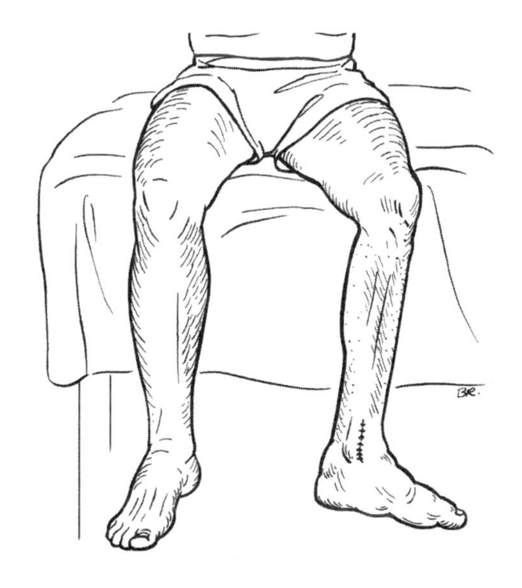

MacGregor (1971) regards deep transverse friction as clinically indispensable. In a paper describing deep friction treatment of medial collateral ligament sprain, coronary ligament sprain, medial meniscus tear, and patellar tendinitis, he suggests that some lesions at the knee are not fully treatable by any other method.

Perhaps its best known proponent is James Cyriax (1977, 1960), who has described the use of deep friction massage in maintaining or restoring painless mobility, claiming that certain lesions – including tendinitis at the shoulder, elbow, hip, knee, and ankle – are incurable by any other means including surgery and steroid infiltration.

According to Cyriax (1984a), properly applied deep friction induces a temporary analgesia that permits treatment to be given which might otherwise be precluded by pain. Schwellnus et al. (1992) found deep transverse frictions to be more effective for reducing pain than a conventional regime of rest, ice, stretching exercises, and ultrasound in the treatment of iliotibial band friction syndrome in athletes.

The therapeutic manipulation itself consists of transverse movements expertly applied either deep into a painful structure or between adherent structures, serving to disrupt

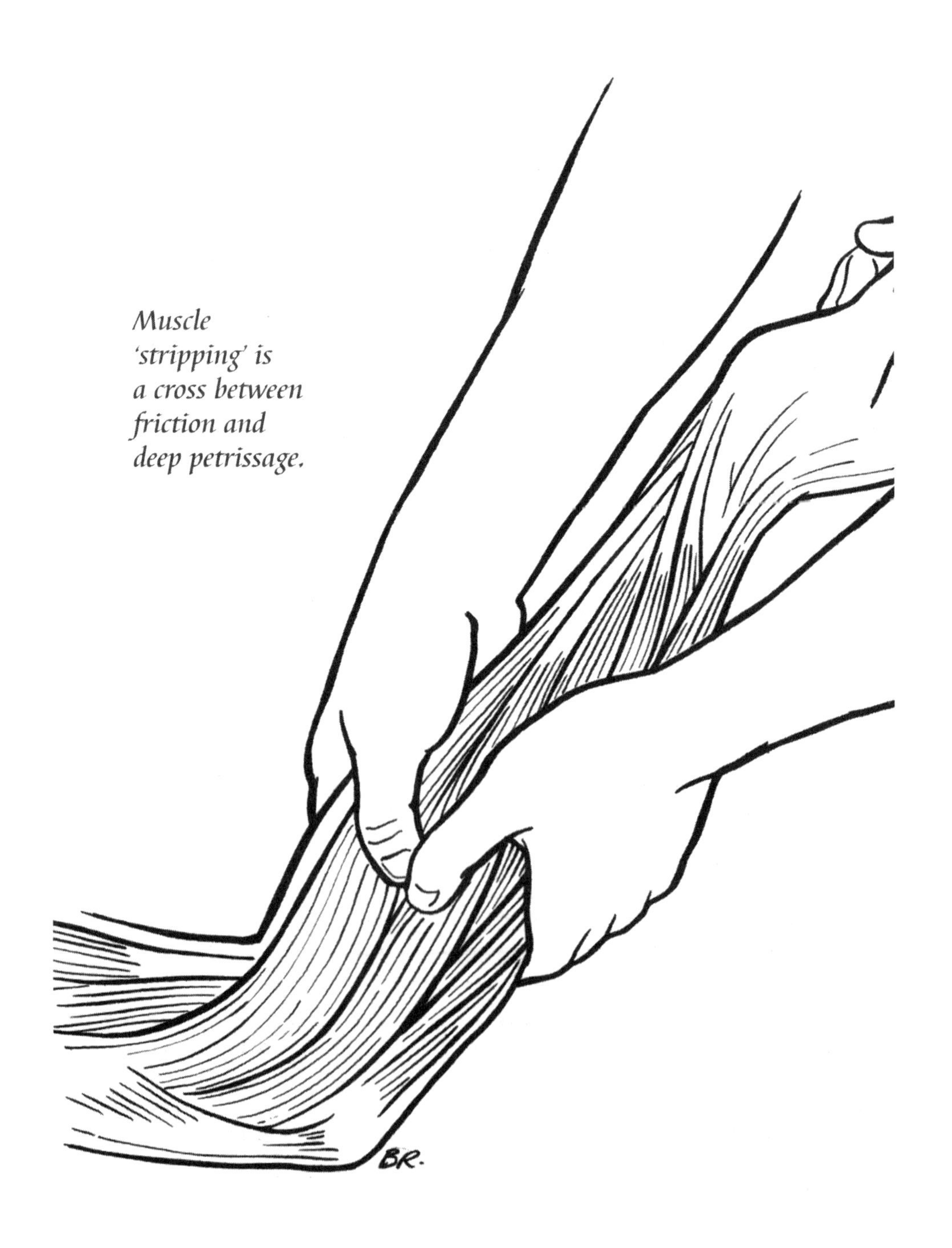

Muscle 'stripping' is a cross between friction and deep petrissage.

both existing and forming adhesions. Transverse friction of a recovering torn ligament, for example, prevents abnormal adherence of the ligament to adjacent bone or connective tissue structures, and encourages optimal internal fiber alignment via normal usage, without causing potentially disruptive stretching of the healing structure.

Treatment Applications

The specific indications for deep friction massage are muscular, tendinous, and ligamentous lesions resulting from recent trauma, although generally not in the acute stage; longstanding scar tissue from old trauma; joints subject to frequent sprains; and acute and chronic tendon disorders such as tendinitis, tenovaginitis, or tenosynovitis (Cyriax, 1984c). Deep friction massage may also be indicated in chronic noncalcific bursitis (Hammer, 1993). In the treatment of these conditions, precisely placed deep transverse frictions are applied for a few minutes at a time to forcibly break adhesions.

- ***Muscular Lesions***

Cyriax (1984a, 1960) asserts that movement restricting adhesions between individual fibers within a muscle cannot be broken by passive stretching or active exercises, but only by forcible broadening of the muscle to separate the linkages. In cases of traumatic injuries undergoing repair, deep friction massage helps prevent the formation of interfibrillary adherences and non-compliant scarring. At old injury sites, transverse frictions disrupt existing adhering and scar tissue that impair expansion of the muscle belly during contraction. Lesions at the musculotendinous junction are, according to Cyriax, untreatable by any other means.

Transverse friction of a recovering torn ligament or tendon prevents abnormal adherence to adjacent bone or connective tissue structures and encourages optimal internal fiber alignment.

- ***Sprains***

Movement of ligaments transversely to the direction of their bony attachments is recommended during recovery from injury, both to prevent adhesions from forming and to break up developing formations. In chronic sprain, the technique is used to eliminate intrinsic and extrinsic adherences that limit elasticity and excursion of the ligament and thus predispose to further sprains (Cyriax 1984c, 1960).

Offering crepitus as proof that gliding surface roughening occurs in tenosynovitis, Cyriax (1960) recommends manual rolling of the tendon sheath to and fro against the tautly held tendon. In a tendon without a sheath, deep friction massage is used to disrupt scar tissue at the tenoperiosteal junction or within the tendon.

Prevention and Treatment of Fibrosis

Askew et al. (1983) studied the effect on hand function of a single treatment session, consisting of paraffin bath, friction massage and active exercise, in ten scleroderma patients. All subjects had improved hand function based on objective measurements and criteria. The authors suggest that regular use of this type of protocol may improve hand function by ameliorating the contracture, loss of strength, and diminished skin compliance commonly associated with scleroderma.

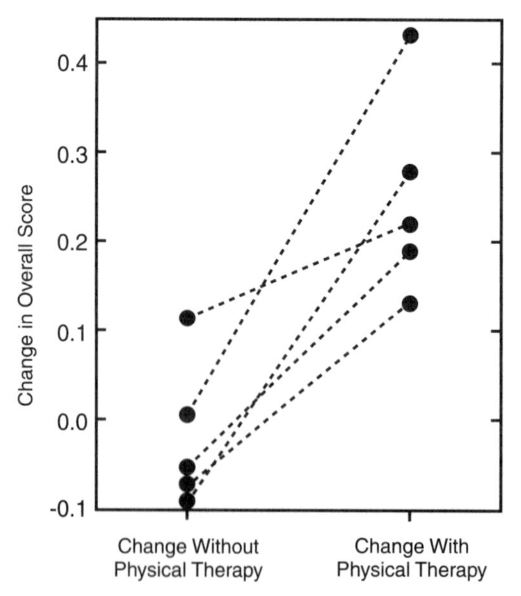

Changes in overall scores of five subjects serving as their own controls.

Askew LJ, et al. Objective Evaluation of Hand Function in Scleroderma Patients to Assess Effectiveness of Physical Therapy, *British Journal of Rheumatology, 1983:22:231, Figure 4.*

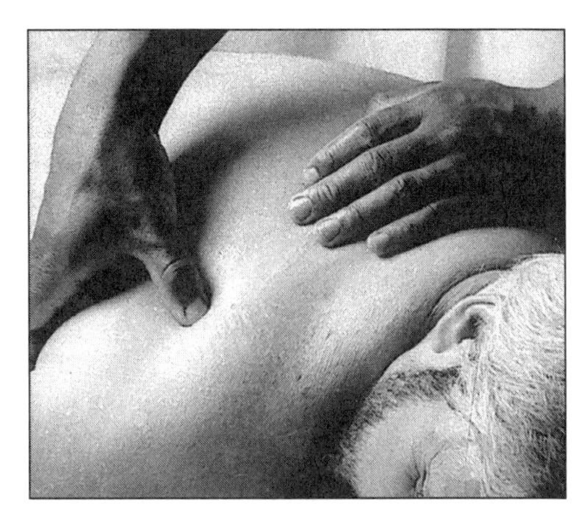

Li (1984) compared 205 cases of frozen shoulder treated by gradual stretching and massage (20 minutes every three days) with 30 cases treated by sudden forced manipulation under nerve block anesthesia followed by daily functional exercises plus massage therapy once every three days. All 205 patients in the first group showed satisfactory improvement, with complete recovery (no pain, function as good as in healthy shoulder) in 71.2 %. Long-term follow-up (1-6 years) of 63 of these individuals showed their recoveries to be sustained. In the group treated with forceful manipulation, complete recovery in terms of pain and function was seen in three cases, and improvement in ten more. Arthroscopic examination revealed evidence of joint capsule rupture in some instances. Li concludes that gradual stretching and massage produce an outcome far superior, in both the short and long term, to that of forced manipulation.

The effectiveness of massage in addressing and preventing fibrosis has also attracted the attention of cosmetic surgeons. Bodian (1969) recommends its use following eyelid surgery and to treat thick scars of the lid, keloid formation, overcorrected entropism, postoperative ectropism, and shallow fornices.

Woodman and Pare (1982) report successful application of deep friction massage in association with steroid injections in treating dancer's heel, Achilles tendinitis, and tenosynovitis of the tibialis posterior and peroneal tendons.

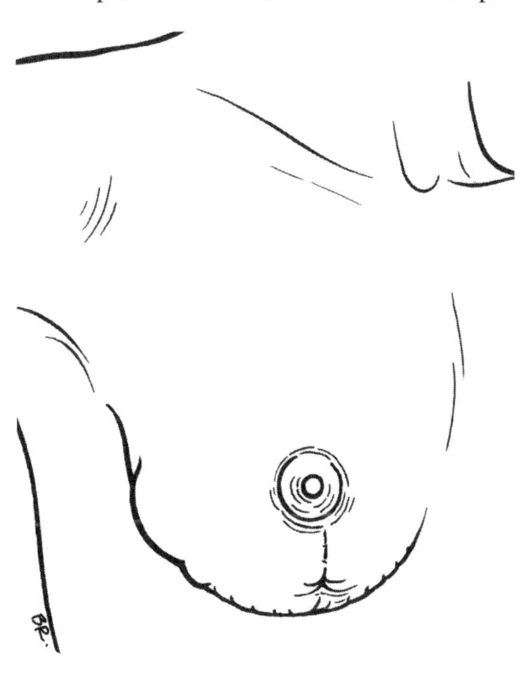

Poor surgical scarring result can be improved with massage therapy.

The value of therapeutic exercise in the treatment of cervical injuries has also been demonstrated. Although for many years the standard protocol for acute neck sprain consisted of rest and immobilization with soft cervical collars, Mealy et al. (1986) have shown that active treatment (using repetitive passive mobilizations and active exercises performed at home) resulted, at eight weeks, in significantly greater improvement in pain intensity and cervical movement compared to standard treatment. In a similar study designed to assess the long term effect of early mobilization exercises in patients with acute neck sprains, McKinney (1989) found that advice to mobilize in the early phase after neck injury reduced symptoms at two years, while prolonged wearing of a collar was associated with persistence of symptoms. Following a review of the currently available literature, the Quebec Task Force on Spinal Disorders (1987) also concluded that active exercise as a part of a multimodal treatment program is beneficial in both the short and the long terms.

The effectiveness of massage in addressing and preventing fibrosis has also attracted the attention of cosmetic surgeons.

Athletic trainers frequently comment on the value of massage therapy in injury rehabilitation and prevention of fibrosis. Although there are few controlled clinical studies of its use in athletics, anecdotal evidence abounds. Matusezewski (1985), in a discussion of massage utilization in athletic training programs, credits it with prevention of fibrosis and adhesions, and loosening and stretching of tight tendons. Further evidence is provided by Harris (1986), who quotes U.S. Olympic competitor Joan Hansen as saying that "an Achilles tendinitis that used to require six weeks of intense physical therapy now only requires five treatments of cross-fiber massage to completely heal the problem."

Indications for Massage Therapy

Some examples of conditions most commonly referred to qualified massage therapists for prevention/treatment of fibrosis and contracture are:

- ***tendinitis, tenovaginitis, tenosynovitis***
- ***muscle strain***
- ***contusions (post acute)***
- ***ligamentous sprain***
- ***iliotibial band syndrome***
- ***painful or non-compliant scar tissue***
- ***torticollis***
- ***whiplash***
- ***compression syndromes and chronic neuralgias***
- ***temporomandibular joint syndrome***
- ***adhesive capsulitis***
- ***post-fracture rehabilitation***
- ***osteoarthritis***

Other conditions for which massage therapy can be similarly beneficial include:

- ***enhancement of post-surgical healing***
- ***Dupuytren's contracture***
- ***degenerative disc disease***
- ***chronic neuritis***
- ***rheumatoid arthritis and other inflammatory conditions of connective tissue***
- ***muscular dystrophy***
- ***myasthenia gravis***
- ***CNS motor disorders such as multiple sclerosis, parkinsonism, and cerebral palsy***

Vibrations

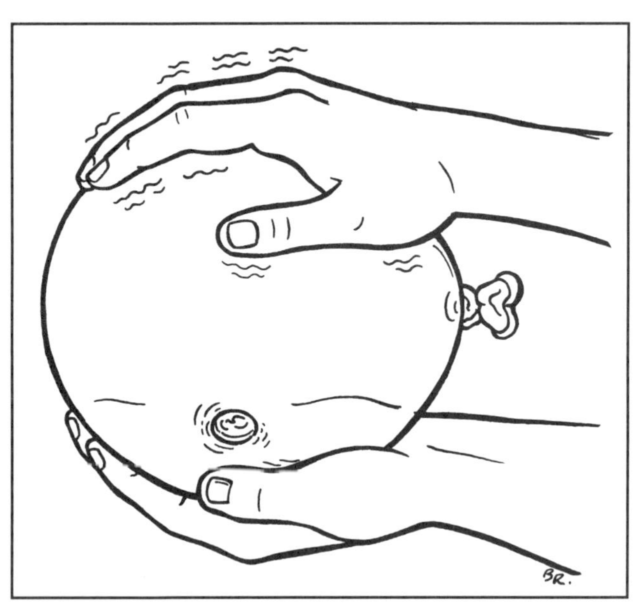

The skill of vibrations is difficult to master. A common practice method involves vibrating a coin inside a balloon without causing any movement of the balloon.

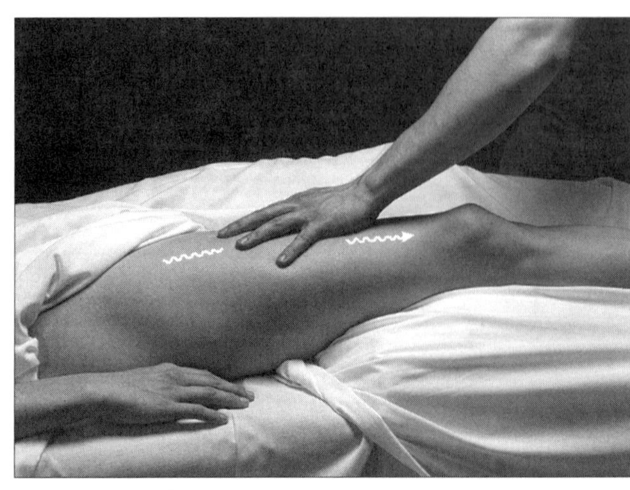

Running Vibrations

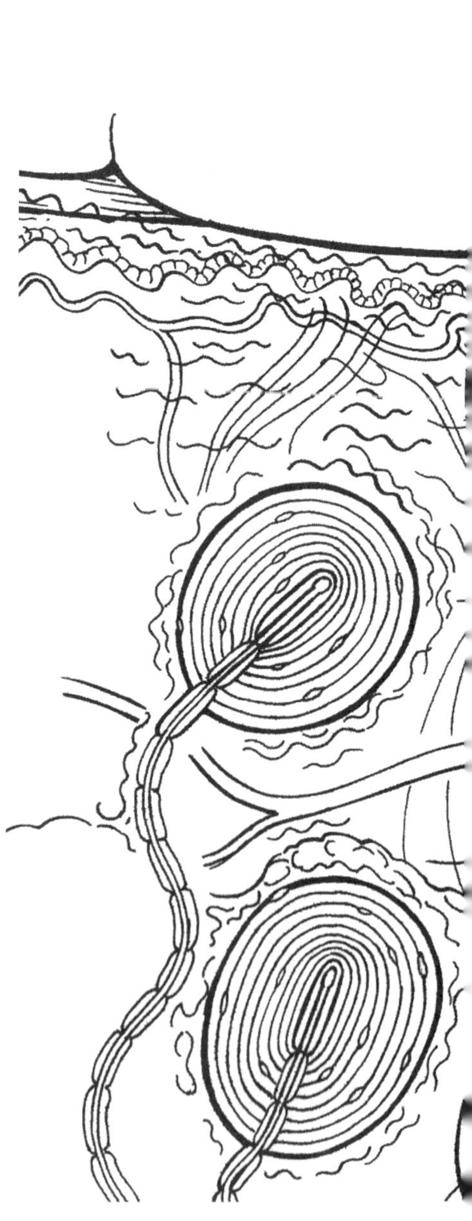

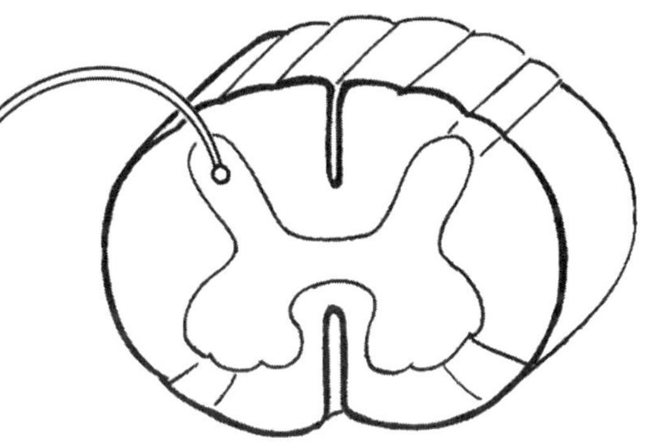

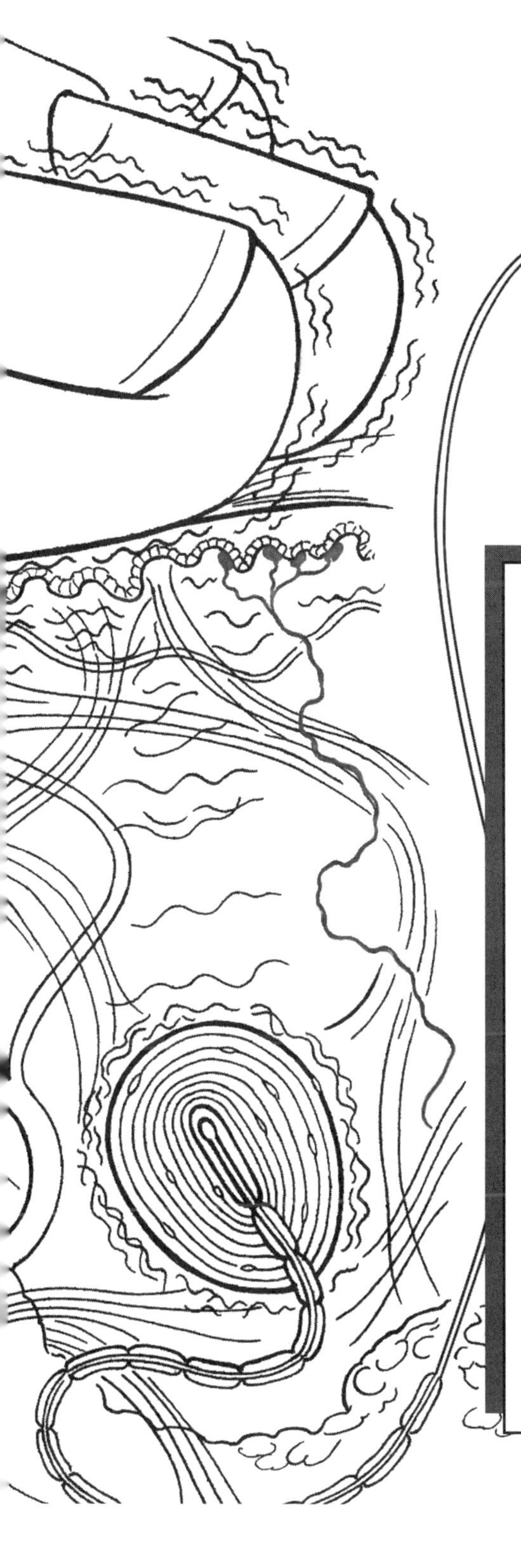

Vibrations Light Reflex Technique

Can be applied in forms that are fine or coarse, with the therapist's hand static or 'running.'

Customary Uses

Fine Vibrations

- Produce a relaxing/calming/soothing effect
- Can create counterirritant analgesia of significant duration
- Used to reflexly reduce muscle tone

Coarse Vibrations

- Produce a mild stimulating effect
- Used to reflexly increase muscle tone e.g. following cast removal
- Used over abdomen to stimulate peristalsis
- Applied over the thorax to loosen respiratory mucus

Avoid (AV) or Adapt For (AD)

AV: Direct use over open or contagious skin lesions
AV: If aggravates pain, e.g. acute injuries
AV: Spasticity
AD: May aggravate asthma

5 Control of Pain

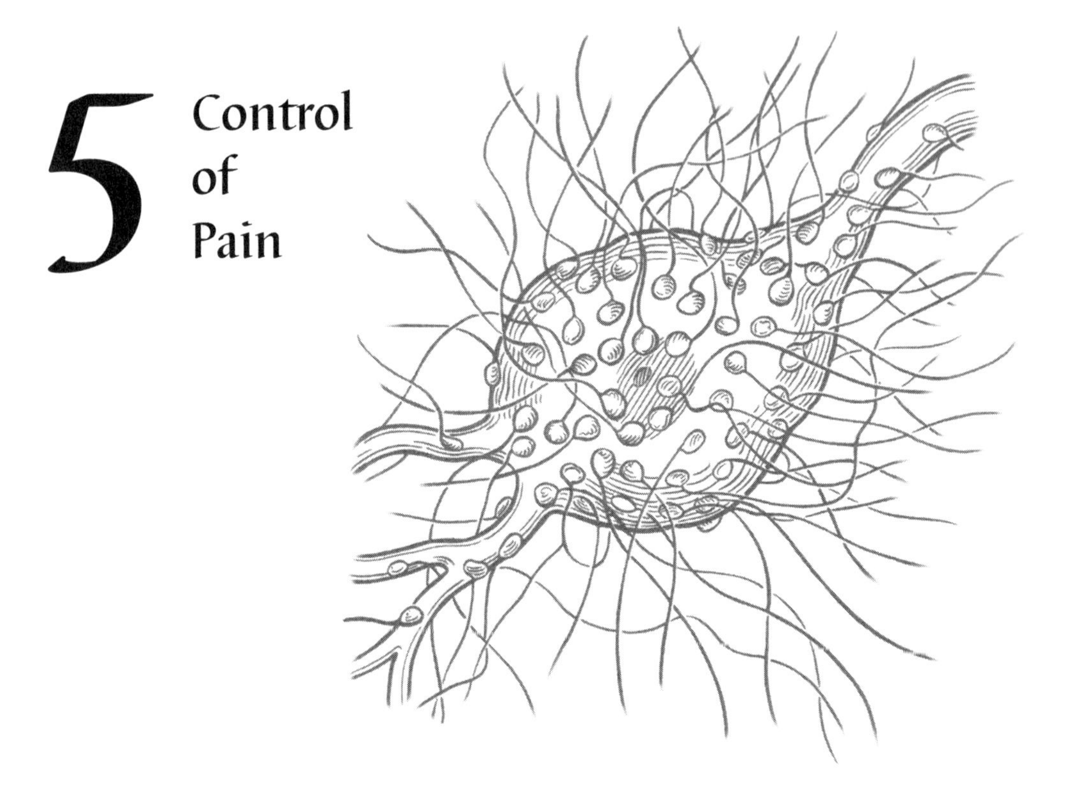

From the intuitive rubbing of a painful injury to the sophisticated application of massage therapy in the treatment of intractable chronic pain, the effectiveness of massage in pain control is widely acknowledged. The report of the Quebec Task Force on Spinal Disorders (1987) states that massage may be the most frequently used therapy for musculoskeletal disorders, and makes particular reference to its usefulness in controlling pain. Breakey (1982) suggests that massage of intensive care and post-surgical patients can decrease the amount of medication required for pain modulation.

There is no shortage of clinical studies and case reports suggesting the far-reaching applicability of massage in pain management. In a randomized controlled trial, Taylor et al. (2003) found that gentle Swedish massage applied post-operatively improves affective and sensory pain and distress in women following abdominal laparotomy. Inagaki et al. (2002) report that 15 minutes of massage and shiatsu provide relief from pain. De Bruijn (1984) applied deep transverse friction to soft tissue injuries in various locations in 13 patients, 11 of whom had tenoperiosteal lesions. Friction massage of 0.4 to 5.1 (mean 2.1) minutes duration resulted in analgesia lasting from 0.3 minutes to 48 hours (mean 26 hours). The author considered the technique clinically important because of its ability to prevent adhesion formation as well as produce analgesia, which permits more functional use of the injured structures.

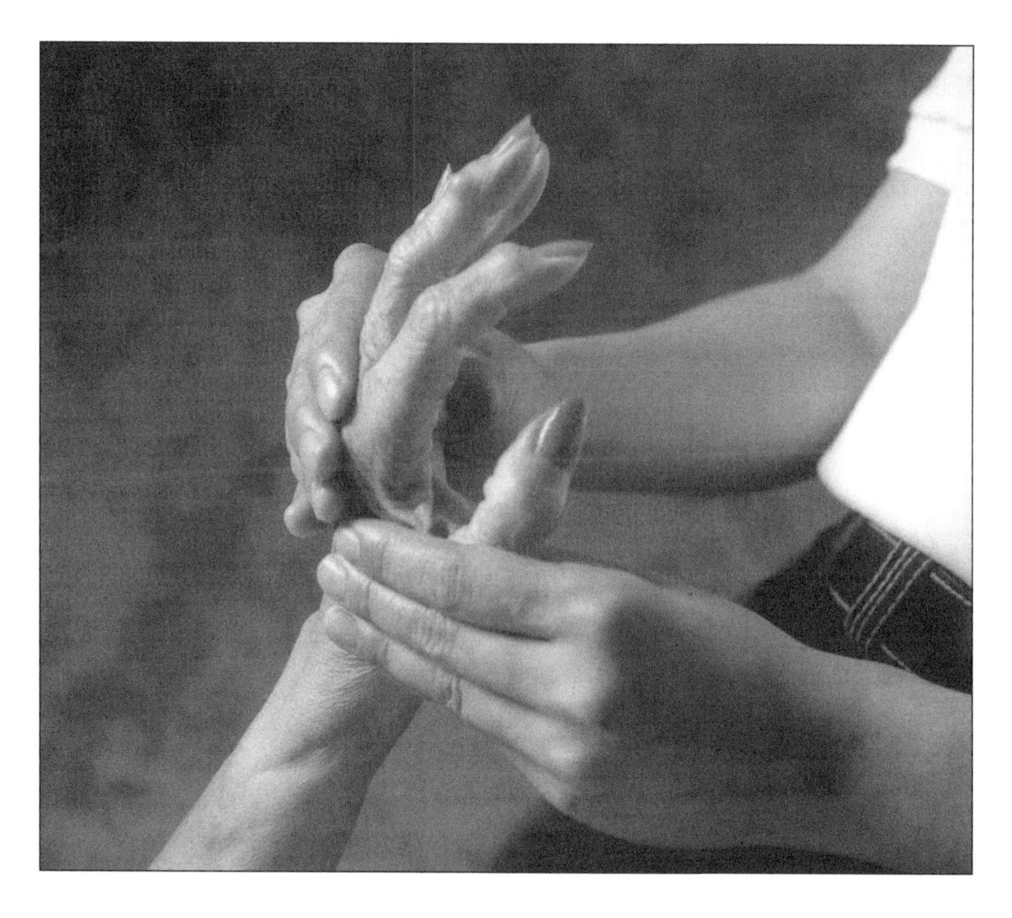

In a case report, Frazer (1978) describes how connective tissue massage (CTM), given according to Ebner's (1975) technique for 20 minutes two or three times a week, proved much more effective than more sophisticated medical treatments for a patient with severe intractable pain following limb sympathectomy.

Another case study by Marshall (1971) reports that a patient with chronic pain achieved complete relief for the first time in 12 months with only two treatments of ice massage. In this case, the patient's spouse was instructed in the technique to deal with recurrences.

Simkin and O'Hara (2002) did a systematic review of five nonpharmacologic childbirth interventions and concluded that massage shows evidence of effectiveness in reducing labor pain and improving other obstetric outcomes. Chang et al. (2002) determined by means of a randomized controlled trial that massage can help decrease pain and anxiety during labor.

Massage therapy is widely used in the treatment of low back pain and some studies have been undertaken to assess its effectiveness. Preyde (2000) described a randomized controlled trial in which patients with subacute low back pain were shown to benefit from massage therapy, and Cherkin et al. (2001) in another randomized trial concluded that therapeutic massage is effective for persistent low back pain. Also, a recent survey by Wolsko et al. (2003) found that 66% of general public respondents found massage to be 'very helpful' in treatment of back and neck pain as compared to 27% for conventional therapies. Although promising evidence has emerged from these studies, several reviewers have pointed out the need for more and better research to confirm their conclusions (Cherkin et al. 2003; Ernst 2003; Furlan et al. 2000; Ernst 1999).

Initiation of reflex muscle contraction in response to nociceptive input is a phenomenon found throughout the somatic neuromuscular system.

There have also been a number of studies demonstrating the value of massage as an adjunct treatment for patients with cancer pain. Smith et al. (2002) found that massage therapy improved scores in pain, sleep quality, and symptom distress as compared both to baseline and to a comparison group not receiving massage. Various forms of treatment including foot massage (Grealish et al. 2000) and massage applied to other parts of the body (Wilkie et al. 2000; Ferrell-Torry & Glick 1993) have been found to reduce pain perception in cancer patients. These changes correlated with improvements in anxiety and stress levels. If there are beneficial changes in pain perception and pain tolerance other than those secondary to decreased anxiety and/or depression, generalized mood improvement, and enhanced sense of well-being, they are inherently difficult to isolate and measure. Such general therapeutic benefits are addressed in Chapters 1 and 7.

The discussion that follows examines what is either known or theorized about specific physiological mechanisms through which massage therapy modifies pain. There are three principal ways in which massage may be expected to achieve pain reduction:

- it may act directly on the source of the pain to alleviate nociceptive[1] stimulation

[1] *Nociception is sensory afferent transmission from distressed tissues that usually proceeds to the brain to be interpreted as pain.*

- it may act centrally to alter the processing of nociceptive input
- it may affect the conduction of pain impulses in the peripheral nerves (least likely of the three, but possibly the mechanism by which local ice massage works)

Alleviation of Nociceptive Input

Muscle pain can arise from prolonged muscle contraction compressing blood vessels within the muscle. Thus the pain associated with spasm or sustained contraction is ischemic pain, which can become part of a pain-contraction cycle.

Jacobs (1960) reviewed the work of Simons et al. (1948), who found that when pain was produced experimentally in a restricted focus in the head area, a secondary, more generalized headache developed that could outlast and exceed the primary triggering pain. Procedures that increased electrical activity in the neck musculature caused an intensification of the headache, implicating sustained contractions of head and neck muscles as a likely source of the secondary pain. Such contractions probably represent a reflex response to the initial painful stimulus, similar to the muscle spasm that produces protective fixation of fractures and sprains. Chronic imbalances of neck and spinal musculature (e.g., in poor posture), sustained concentration (e.g., prolonged use of the eyes), and emotional tension may also result in headache.

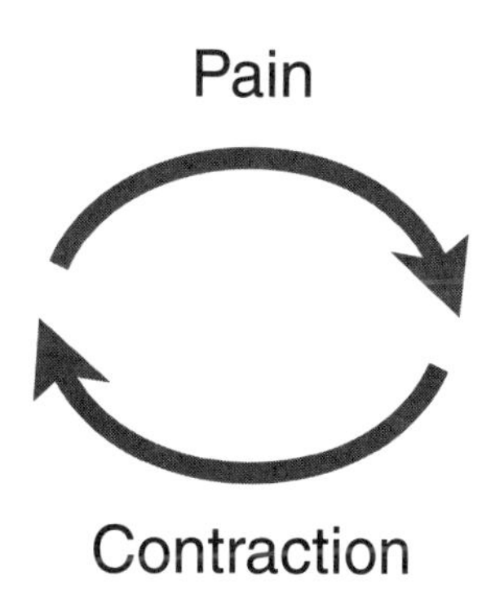

Initiation of reflex muscle contraction in response to nociceptive input is a phenomenon found throughout the somatic neuromuscular system, so it is not unreasonable to extrapolate this head pain scenario to other parts of the body. In the case of backache, for example, even when the primary local cause is minimal, reflex muscle contraction and muscle tension from anxiety and emotional distress may cause secondary back pain that outlasts and exceeds the primary discomfort.

According to Jacobs (1960), the therapeutic effect of massage in such syndromes is associated with breaking the pain-contraction cycle. This can be accomplished through improved circulation in venous and lymphatic channels (possibly assisted by release of vasodilators like histamine) and through reflex dilation of vessels through stimulation of the cutaneous afferents mediating touch and pressure. Relaxation of contracted or spasmed muscles also results from stimulation of proprioceptors in the muscle, tendon, joint capsule, and fascia via stretching and compressive movements.

It is possible that the effectiveness of massage in treating myofascial trigger points and relieving their referred pain phenomena may also be partly explained in terms of interrupting a pain-contraction cycle.

Alteration of Central Processing of Nociceptive Input

Our understanding of the CNS mechanisms by which pain sensations are modified has been greatly expanded in recent years by the theory of neural gating (Watson 1981a; Melzack & Wall 1965), and by the discovery of a brain analgesic system involving neurons in the brainstem and dorsal horns of the spinal cord (Watson 1981b; Basbaum & Fields 1978). Both have been suggested as possible explanations for the achievement of analgesia through massage. The neural gating mechanism has been used to explain modification of pain transmission via the large sensory afferent inputs created by acupuncture, acupressure, and electrical currents (Goats 1990; Melzack et al. 1980a), as well as by massage (Bowsher 1988), CTM (Goats & Keir 1991), and joint manipulation (Grieve 1981). More recently, Lund et al. (2002) reported that massage-like stroking induces short-term antinociceptive effects in rodents. Long-term results, evidenced by increased hind-paw withdrawal latencies after six every-other-day treatments, continued to increase over the observation period, which included seven additional treatments. The effects were reversed by an oxytocin antagonist, indicating a role for oxytocin in endogenous pain control systems, and suggesting another piece in the explanation of massage's antinociceptive effects.

The neural gating mechanism has been used to explain modification of pain transmission via the large sensory afferent inputs created by massage, CTM and joint manipulation.

The Quebec Task Force on Spinal Disorders (1987) suggested that elevation of endorphin levels in the CNS as a result of massage could be an important mechanism in pain modulation. Day et al. (1987) sought to provide objective information about this by measuring plasma beta-endorphin and beta-lipoprotein levels in normal, pain free subjects before and after a 30 minute back massage. No significant changes were found. While it does not appear that massage increases endogenous opiate production in normal individuals, the possibility remains that this mechanism plays some role when pain is present. In particular, responses on the psychological level may act via this mechanism, for example confidence in the therapist and the treatment may lead to increased activity of the brain analgesic system. It does appear that relaxing massage increases tolerance for therapies producing discomfort (Simpson 1991), for post-operative pain (Nixon et al. 1997), and for pain associated with fibromyalgia (Sunshine et al. 1996), juvenile rheumatoid arthritis (Field et al. 1997a), burn injuries (Field et al. 1998a), and cancer (Ferrell-Tory & Glick 1993).

On the other hand, the deep direct pressure of CTM has been found to result in moderate beta-endorphin release lasting for about an hour (Kaada & Torsteinbo 1989). Goats (1994) suggests that other treatments that cause discomfort will act in a similar manner, including vigorous conventional massage, transverse frictions, and certain percussive techniques. One of the benefits of deep friction massage in the treatment of soft tissue injuries is the temporary analgesia it produces, which permits otherwise painful mobilizations and therapeutic exercises to be performed (Cyriax 1984a; Swezey 1983). Although the explanation usually offered for this analgesia is activation of the neural gating mechanism in the spinal cord through stimulation of large fiber proprioceptors and cutaneous mechanoreceptors, release of endorphins and enkephalins may also be involved. It has also been suggested (Swezey 1983) that stimulation of proprioceptive nerve endings by focal deep pressure and massage over trigger points facilitates enkephalin release and pain modulation in the spinal cord, thus helping to interrupt the pain-contraction cycle.

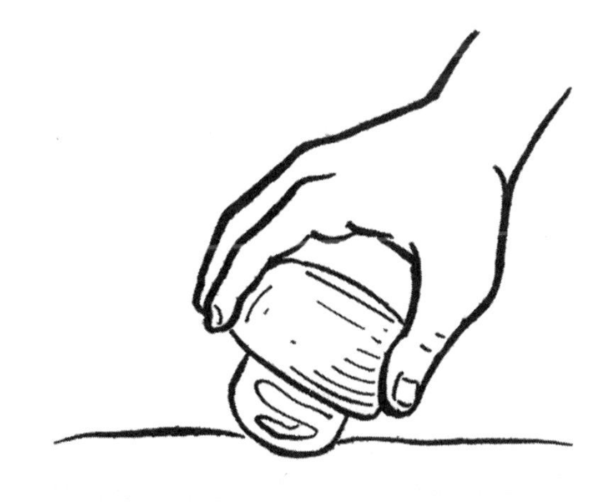

Ice Massage

Several studies indicate that, like acupuncture and Transcutaneous Electrical Nerve Stimulation (TENS), ice massage activates the pain gating system in the spinal cord. Melzack et al. (1980a) found that ice massage and TENS

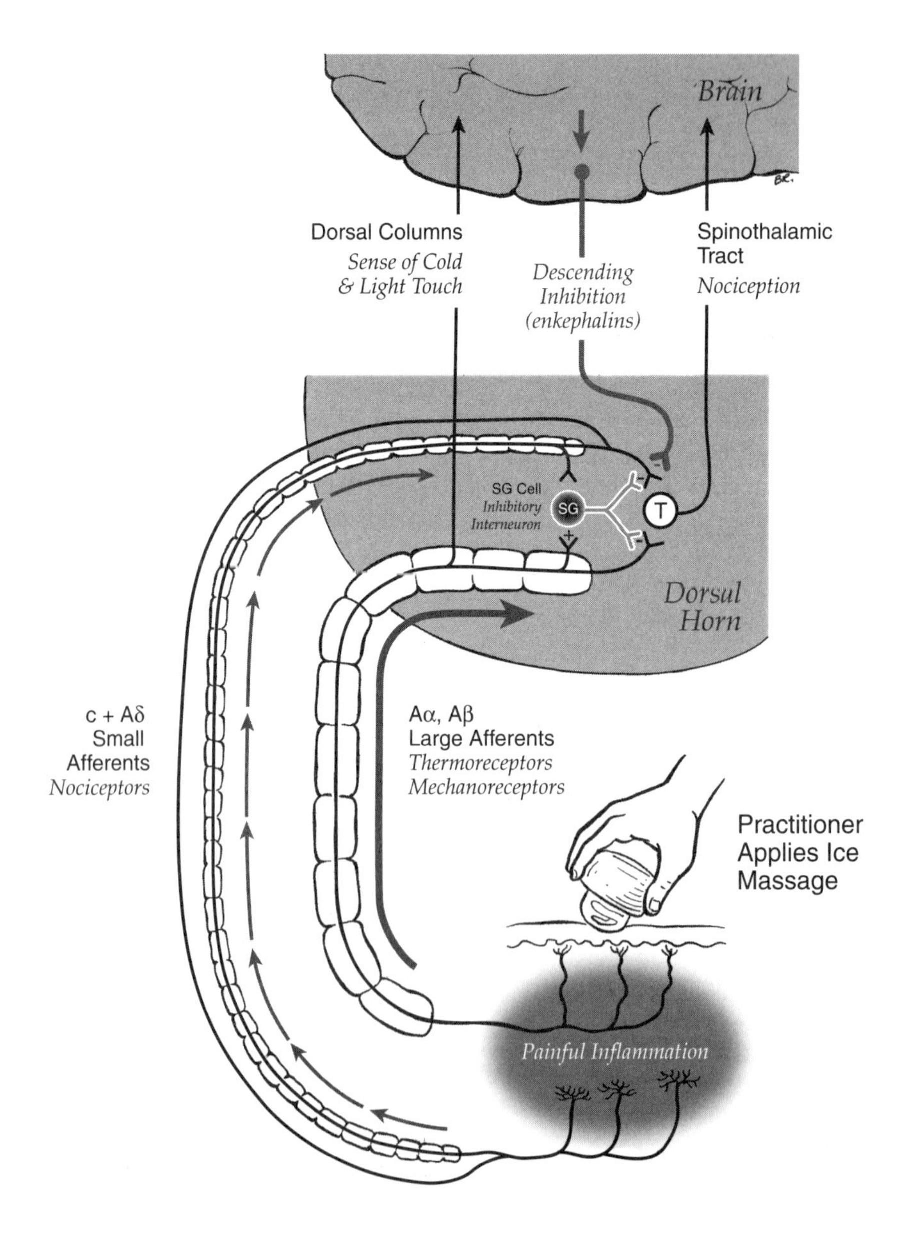

According to the neural gating theory, stimuli such as temperature and touch close the pain 'gate' by reaching the dorsal horn before slower nociceptive transmission, suggesting, at least in part, an explanation of how massage reduces pain sensation.

applied to the same locations (the midline of the back at L3 and S1 and the lateral malleolus) were equally effective in relieving low back pain; ice massage appeared to be more effective than TENS for some patients.

In a study of patients with dental pain (Melzack et al. 1980b), ice massage was applied to the web between the thumb and index finger on the same side of the body as the pain. Pain intensity decreased by more than 50% in most subjects. Similar results were obtained by Melzack & Bentley (1983) in patients with acute dental pain, the intensity of which was decreased 40-50% after ice massage of the ipsilateral hand or contralateral hand or arm (treatment of the ipsilateral arm produced no significant result).

> *Ice massage was found to be effective in achieving analgesia sufficient to permit therapeutic exercise. Reduced nerve conduction velocity was the explanation given for the analgesic effect.*

The analgesic effect of ice massage in these examples cannot be explained in terms of either eliminating the source of the pain or blocking pain impulse conduction through nerve fiber cooling. Because the pain-relieving effects demonstrated for ice massage are comparable to those of TENS and acupuncture, it is possible that all three share the same underlying neural mechanism involving the gating of pain within the spinal cord.

Peripheral Conduction of Pain Impulses

Massage may also alleviate pain through direct effects on peripheral nerves. In a review of ice massage for management of acute neuromuscular pain, Waylonis (1967) suggests that its physiological effects are similar to those produced by other cooling methods such as ethyl chloride spray, ice packs, and cold water. These effects are commonly thought to include a reduction in local circulation and metabolism, lessening the generation of nociceptive impulses and decreasing the rate of conduction of peripheral nerve impulses (Murphy 1959; Bierman 1955).

According to early work by Denny-Brown et al. (1945), effective blocking of nerve conduction occurs in sensory fibers at temperatures below 10ºC. More recently, Bugaj (1975) found that analgesia was elicited by ice massage once the area had been cooled to and maintained below a skin temperature of 13.6ºC. A ten minute ice massage was found to be effective in achieving analgesia sufficient to permit therapeutic exercise. Reduced nerve conduction velocity was the explanation given for the analgesic effect, an effect that previous investigators had found to occur beginning at temperatures below 27ºC. Some question remains about the relative importance of changes in conduction velocity versus changes in receptor metabolism. Wolf (1975), in response to Bugaj's paper, speculated that the analgesia might be due to temporary metabolic changes within cutaneous receptors.

Massage therapy can be very effective in circumstances where fear contributes to the level of discomfort, for example in cancer care and in pediatrics.

Regardless of mechanism, there is little doubt about the efficacy and widespread use of cold in pain management. Grant (1964) and Hayden (1964) report symptomatic improvement in 95% of 7,300 outpatients treated with ice massage in a large military hospital. Travell & Simons (1983) prescribe the use of cold to depress the activity of pain receptors, thereby permitting passive stretching and active exercise in the treatment of myofascial pain.

Indications for Massage Therapy in the Control of Pain

Massage therapy may be useful in pain management for post-trauma and post-surgical patients, cardiac patients, and the terminally ill. It can be very effective in circumstances where fear contributes to the level of discomfort, for example in cancer care and in pediatrics, as well as in situations where medication is insufficient to achieve pain control or causes unacceptable side effects.

Note that pain is also relieved by decreasing circulatory congestion, by alleviating myofascial trigger points, and/or increasing ROM.

Conditions for which massage therapy is commonly used for pain control include:

- ***fibromyalgia***
- ***most types of soft tissue lesions***
- ***pain associated with inflammation and injury recovery***
- ***whiplash and whiplash associated disorder (WAD)***
- ***arthritis and other lesions affecting joints***
- ***overuse and sports related pain syndromes***
- ***painful postural dysfunctions***
- ***neuritis and neuralgia, including trigeminal neuralgia and sciatica***
- ***headache***
- ***temporomandibular joint syndrome***
- ***labor and delivery***
- ***dysmenorrhea***

Tapotement

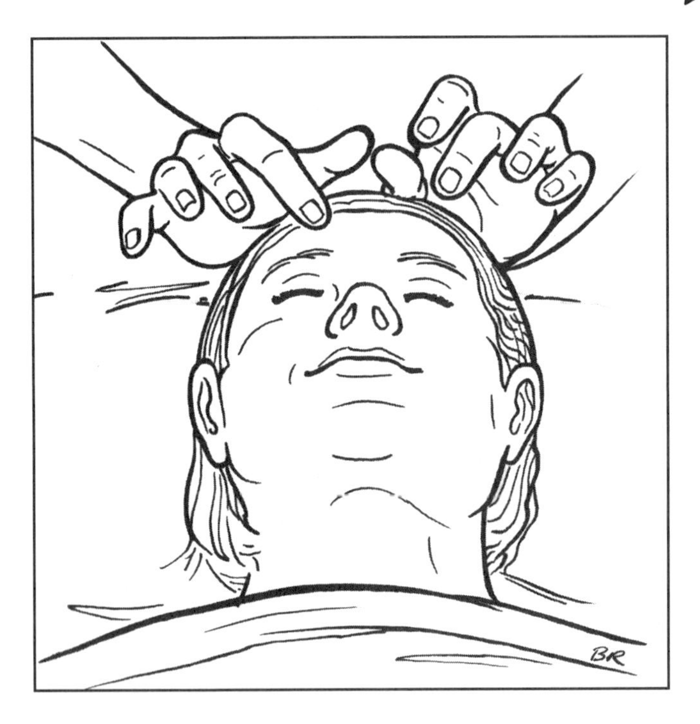

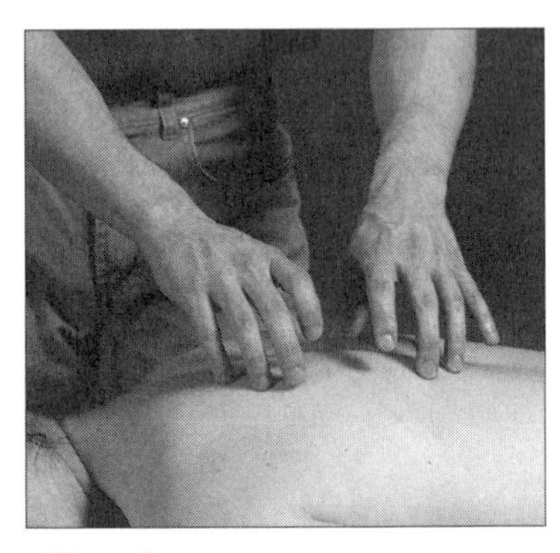
Tapping

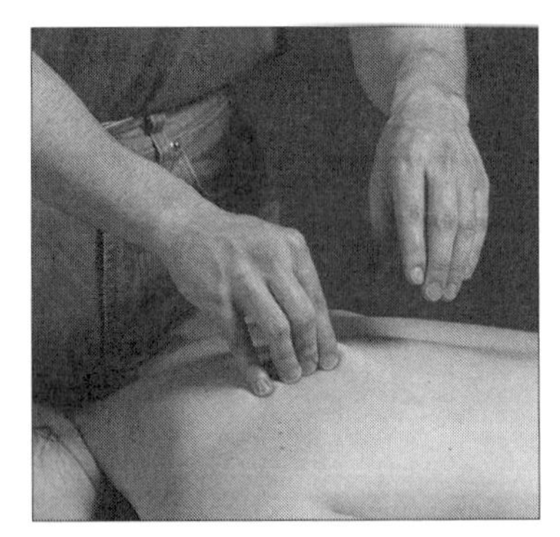
Pincement

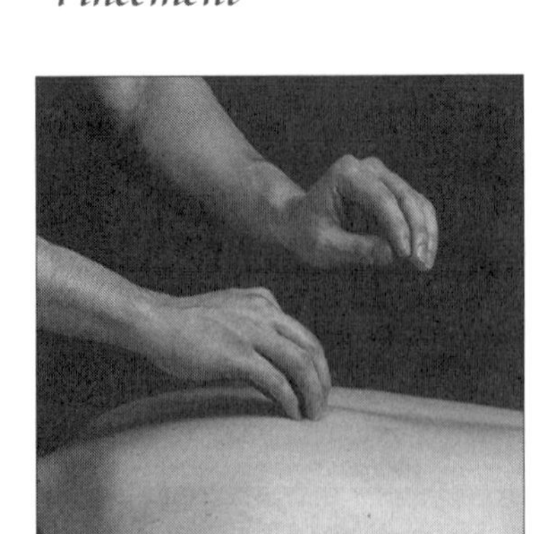
Light Hacking

Light Tapotement

Customary Uses

Reflexly increases muscle tone
(e.g. post-casting, recovering nerve injury)
Helps rehabilitate sensory afferent transmission
Mild sedative effect if used on head, face, back
Stimulates glandular activity of skin

Avoid (AV) or Adapt For (AD)

AV: If aggravates painful condition, irritated tissue
AV: Hypersensitive sensory responses
AV: Spasticity

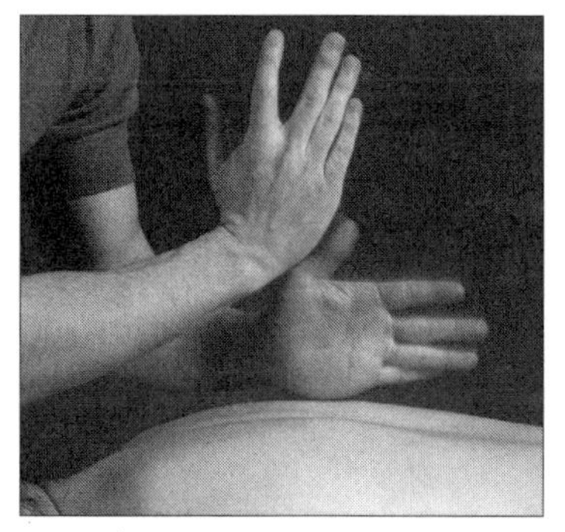

Hacking

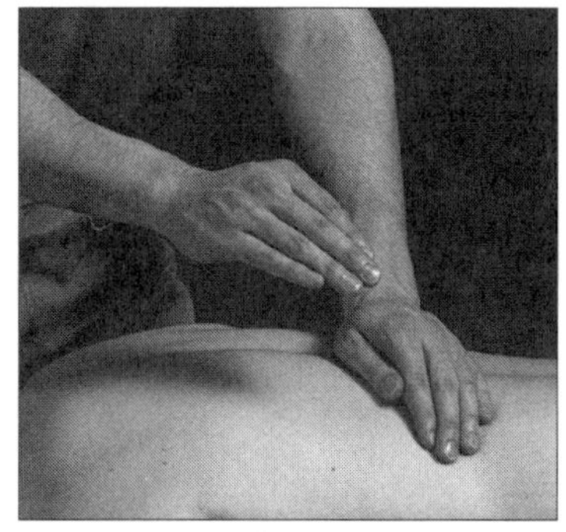

Cupping/Clapping

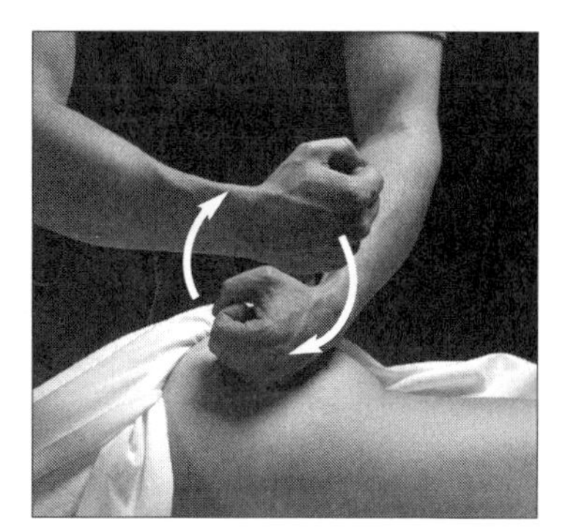

Pounding

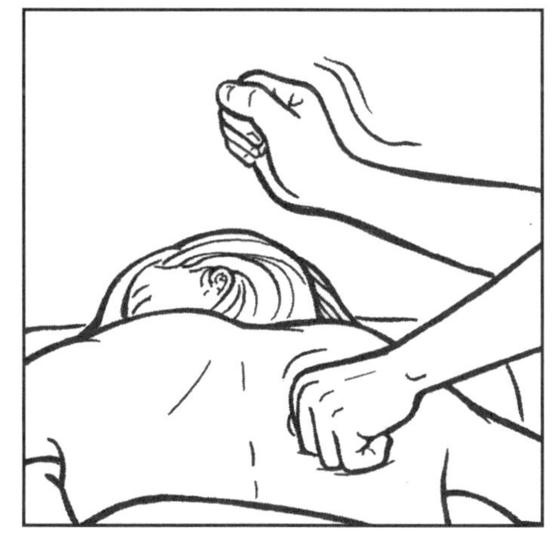

Beating/Rapping

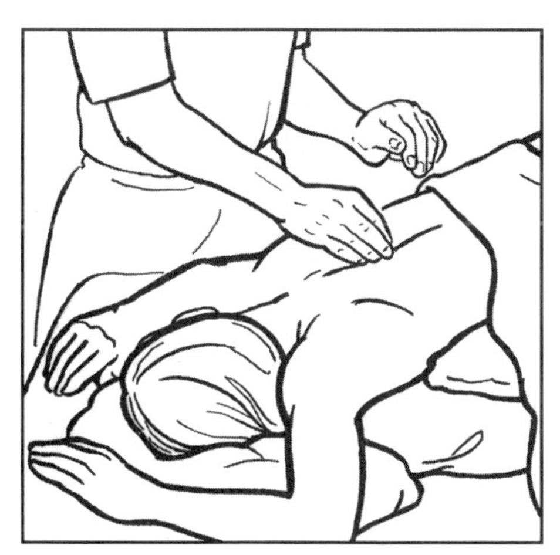

Cupping and Postural Drainage

Heavy Tapotement

Customary Uses

- Increases local circulation, metabolism
- Increases sympathetic activation
  - : Pre- and post-event for athletes
  - : At treatment end, if more alertness is desired
- Temporarily increases muscle tone, followed by secondary relaxation
- Counterirritant analgesia (pain relief, amputations)
- Used over the thorax, loosens mucus and promotes expectoration and coughing

Avoid (AV) or Adapt For (AD)

- AV: Recent fracture or soft tissue injury
- AV: Ribcage injury, radiation induced weaknesses
- AV: Osteoporosis, especially advanced
- AV: Over abdomen, kidneys, bony prominences
- AV: Over sacrum during pregnancy
- AV: Unstable cardiac conditions, dysrhythmia
- AV: Conditions prone to hemorrhage, weakened blood vessels
- AV: Epilepsy
- AV: Neuritis, neuralgia, most painful conditions
- AV: Gastrointestinal reflux
- AV: Over muscle spasm; spasticity
- AV: During asthma attack; may trigger attack
- AD: Hypertension

6 Respiratory Function

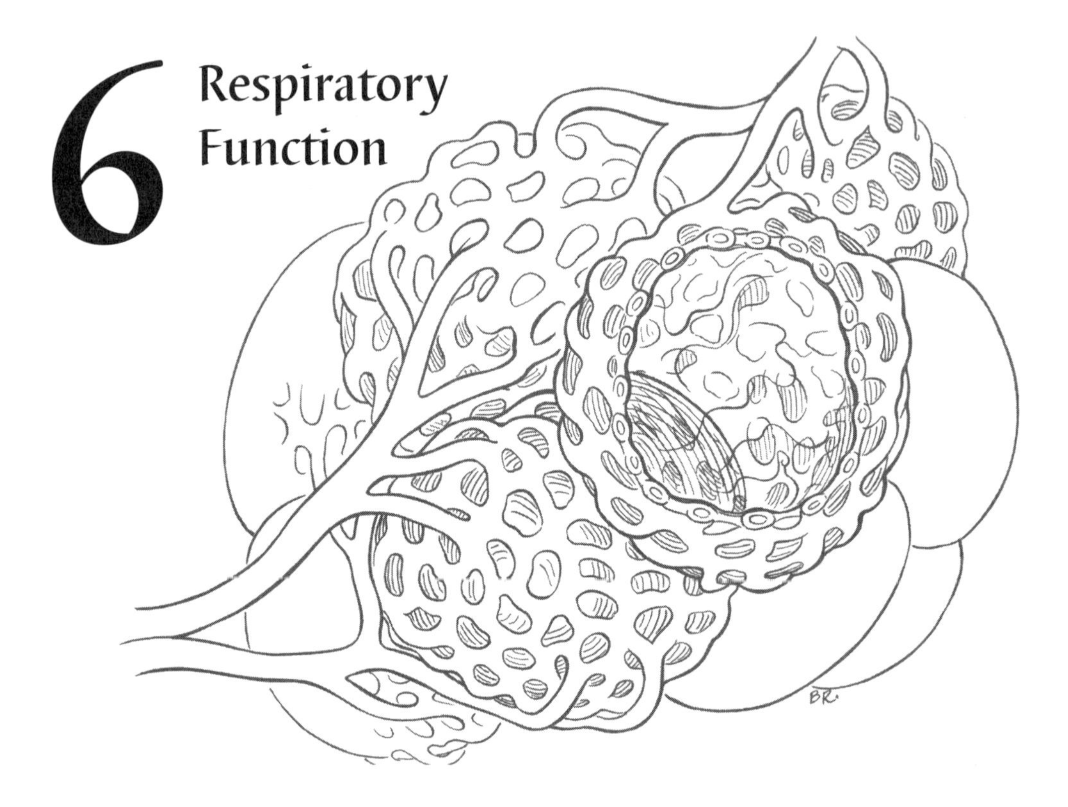

Massage techniques have been used for many years as a component of treatment regimens for patients with respiratory disease. There are two specific therapeutic benefits for which massage therapy is employed:

- increased mucociliary transport with sputum production and improved air flow, produced by means of chest percussions and/or vibration massage, with or without postural drainage
- improved function of the respiratory muscles, which become heavily overtaxed in chronic obstructive lung disease (COPD), through a variety of muscle and connective tissue focused treatment approaches as discussed in Chapters 3 and 4

It can also be noted that increased ease and depth of respiration are an aspect of the general relaxation response induced during massage of both healthy and ill subjects. This type of result is broadly reported in studies of massage therapy outcomes such as those represented in Chapter 1. Relaxation-based effects can be expected to contribute to the massage therapy benefits experienced by individuals with respiratory disease.

Percussion, Vibration and Postural Drainage

Percussion, vibration and postural drainage techniques have been core treatment approaches since the pre-war era when physical therapy and massage therapy were closely interrelated, and they persist in the treatment regimens of both disciplines for conditions of respiratory congestion.

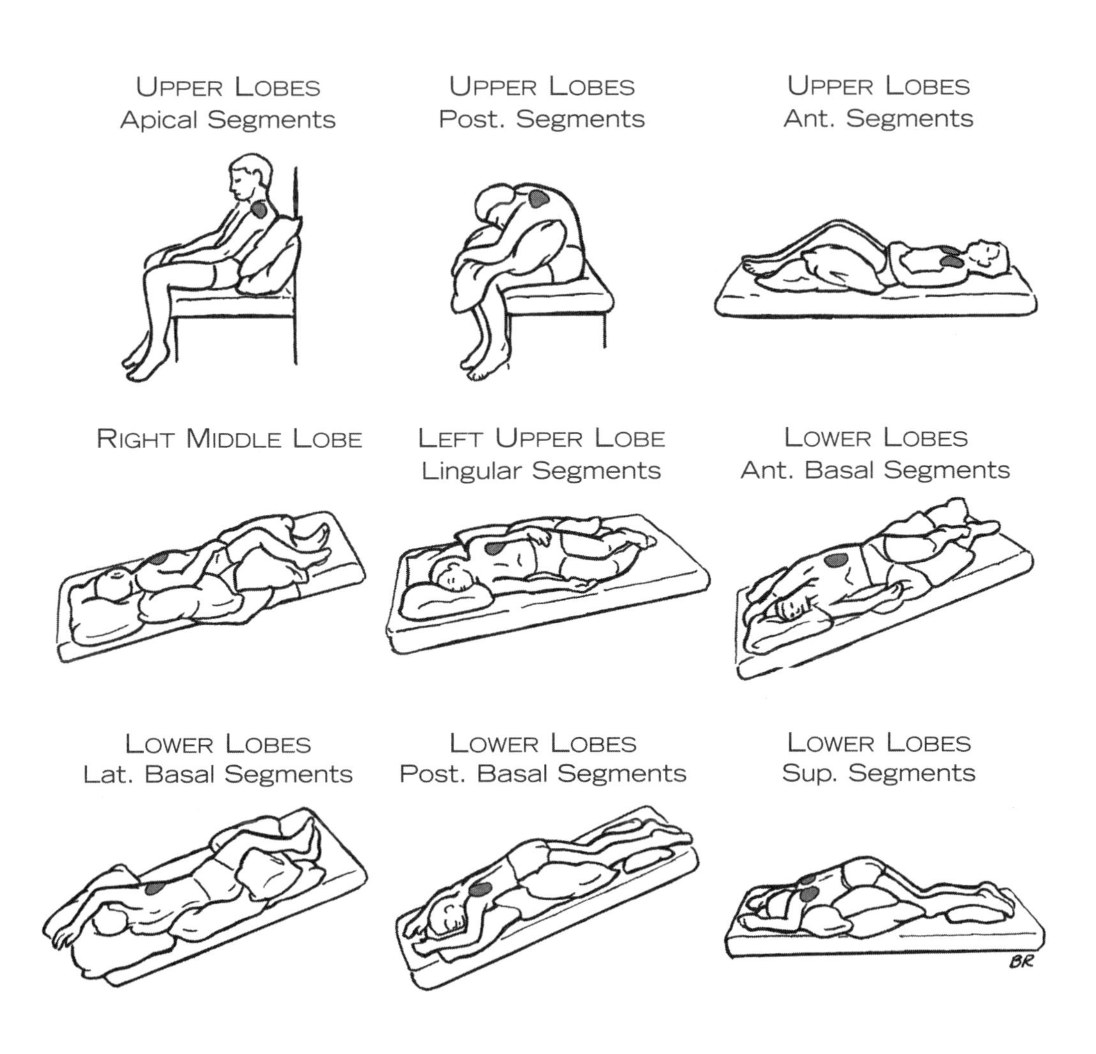

Postural Drainage Positions

Percussion and vibration loosen secretions to enhance the rate of mucociliary transport in the airways (Andrade & Clifford 2001). Postural drainage utilizes gravity to also enhance airway transport and clearance. Chopra et al. (1977) measured tracheal transport velocity in dogs using a radioactive tracer. Transport velocity was found to increase by 50.9% with chest percussion and 39.7% with postural drainage, which, together with hydration, are the physical measures commonly employed for COPD. The authors refer to a paper by Pham et al. (1973), who report that vibration, percussion, and postural drainage significantly decreased sputum viscosity and improved arterial PO_2 and alveolar-arterial PO_2 difference in 38 patients with chronic bronchitis. They also cite a study by Clarke et al. (1973), who found an improvement in one-second forced expiratory volume (FEV_1) and specific airway conductance in twenty-three subjects treated by the same methods. Dallimore et al. (1998) report that oxygen saturation was increased with percussion during quiet breathing in seven healthy subjects.

Postural drainage combined with percussion is generally found to be more effective than postural drainage alone, although percussion is sometimes associated with a slight transient (<20 minutes) decrease in FEV_1. This decrease is suggested to be due to bronchospasm, but may also be the direct and immediate result of disturbing mucous secretions within the airways (Irwin & Tecklin, 1995; Campbell et al. 1975).

A recent study (Doering et al. 1999) was conducted on the influence of manual vibratory massage on the pulmonary function of postoperative patients who were receiving mechanical ventilation following heart or lung transplantation. Significant improvements were seen in mean tidal volume (30% increase), central venous pressure (11% decrease), and pulmonary vessel resistance (18.3% decrease), all of which contributed to improved ventilation/perfusion ratios. The authors suggest that these results may be due to both increased mucociliary clearance and a relaxing effect on the respiratory muscles. Another study by Hammon et al. (1993) compared manual chest percussion to mechanical chest percussion for removing proteinaceous material from the alveoli of patients with pulmonary alveolar proteinosis. The authors conclude that manual percussion is superior to mechanical percussion in increasing the therapeutic results of whole-lung bronchopulmonary lavage.

Treatment of the Respiratory Musculature

Chronic lung disease is associated with maladaptive musculoskeletal changes that largely stem from irritation, shortening, and fatigue of respiratory muscles. The accessory muscles, in particular, tend to be overused to assist in routine breathing (Breslin, 1996; Carter & Coast, 1993). When chronic cough is present additional musculoskeletal stresses occur. Altered recruitment and over-recruitment of respiratory

Muscles of Respiration

Primary Inhalation
Diaphragm
External Intercostals

Accessory Inhalation
Scalenes
Sternocleidomastoid
Subclavius
Serratus Posterior Superior
Pectoralis Major & Minor

Primary Exhalation
None—Passive Process

Accessory Exhalation
Internal Intercostals
Abdominals
Quadratus Lumborum

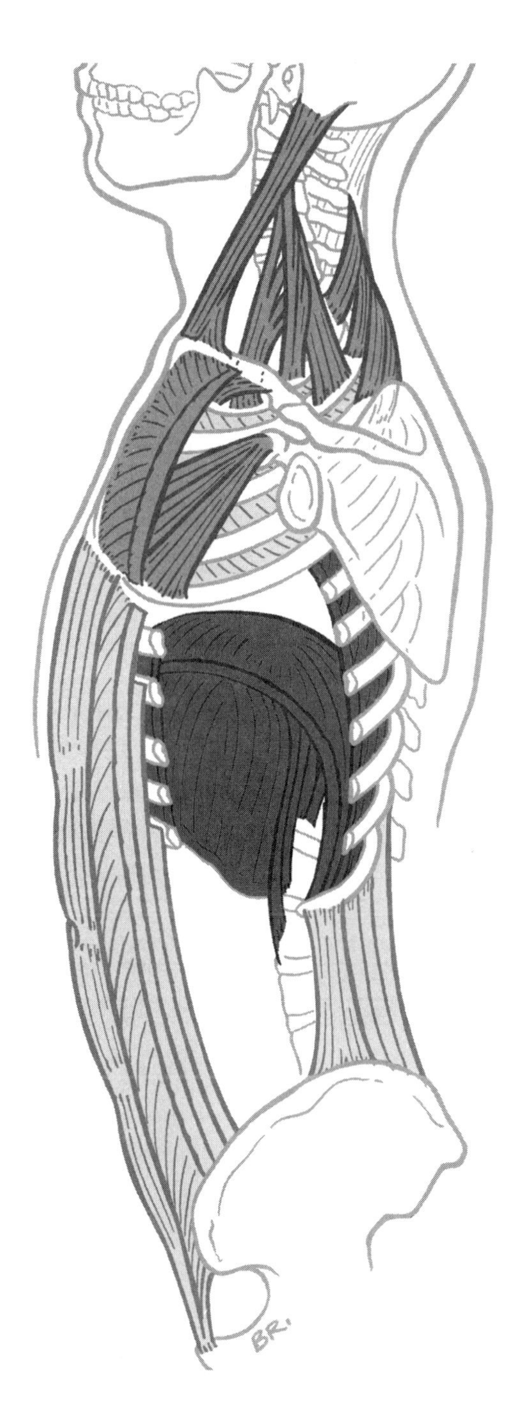

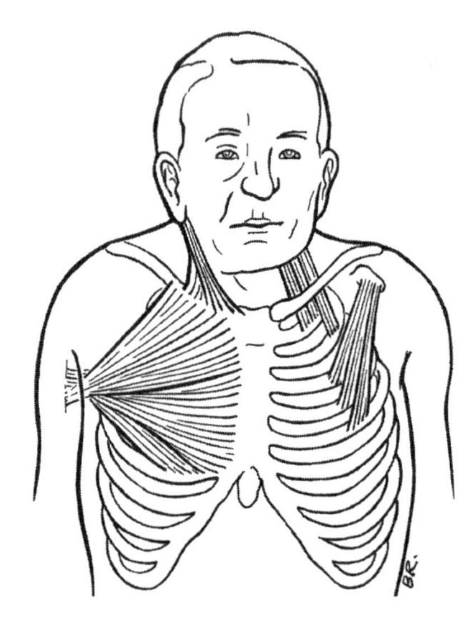

'Barrel Chest'
typical of chronic dyspneic conditions

musculature leads to neck stiffness, decreased rib cage mobility, and dysfunctional thoracic mechanics and postures. A downward cycle sets in, with respiratory muscle fatigue becoming a secondary cause of hypoventilation in COPD patients (Begin & Grassino 1991).

High tension and anxiety levels are also common in individuals with dyspneic respiratory conditions, resulting in a complex cause-and-effect relationship between muscle tension, reduced rib cage mobility, and impaired breathing. Muscles involved in normal and forced respiration include the diaphragm, sternocleidomastoid, external and internal intercostals, scalenes, levator costorum, serratus posterior superior, pectoralis major and minor, quadratus lumborum, and the abdominal wall muscles. Other muscles that may be involved include trapezius, latissimus dorsi, serratus anterior, and iliocostalis lumborum (Rattray et al. 2000).

Witt & MacKinnon (1986) performed four 20-minute sessions of Trager Psychophysical Integration (consisting of gentle painless passive movements of the

TABLE 3
Means and Standard Deviations for the Criterion Measures (N = 12)

Measurement		Pretest	Posttest	Follow-up	*p*
FVC (L)	χ	1.79	2.03	2.01	<.05
	s	0.75	0.67	0.63	
FEV_1/Observed FVC (%)	χ	64.33	57.59	58.16	NS
	s	14.80	24.30	22.13	
FEV_2/Observed FVC (%)	χ	84.30	83.96	90.00	NS
	s	10.70	10.50	14.30	
RR (breaths/min)	χ	17.70	15.70	15.90	<.05
	s	3.60	2.60	4.30	
Chest expansion (cm)	χ	3.60	8.15	5.60	<.06
	s	2.00	2.60	1.90	

Witt PL, MacKinnon J. Trager Psychophysical Integration. A Method to Improve Chest Mobility of Patients with Chronic Lung Disease. *Physical Therapy, 1986; 66:216*

neck, abdomen, and chest wall) on patients with emphysema, bronchitis and asthma, and found significant post-treatment improvement in forced vital capacity, respiratory rate, and chest expansion. FEV_1 at one and three seconds was not significantly changed. Subjective responses to treatment indicated general relaxation and decreases in anxiety and tension. The authors conclude that the technique produces positive effects upon the restrictive component of COPD (the obstructive component did not improve) and particularly recommend that therapists become familiar with the technique.

Beeken et al. (1998) found that 4 out of 5 COPD patients receiving neuromuscular release massage treatment – a combination of myofascial trigger point work and other massage techniques specifically directed towards improving the status of chronically tense and shortened muscles – had increased thoracic gas volume, peak flow, and forced vital capacity. The findings suggest that this type of treatment approach benefits patients with chronic obstructive lung disease, and that the effects may be attributable to improved respiratory muscle function. Field et al. (1998b) also report that massage improves forced expiratory flow and other pulmonary functions in children with asthma.

Respiratory Conditions for which Massage Therapy is Indicated

Massage therapy is indicated in the treatment of individuals with:

- ***asthma***
- ***chronic bronchitis***
- ***emphysema***
- ***other COPDs***
- ***assistance with clearance following respiratory flus and similar common illnesses***
- ***following surgery where respiratory structures are affected***

Management of these conditions would involve a situation-specific selection of treatment approaches including general relaxation and anxiety reduction, chest percussion, vibration and postural drainage, and treatment of the respiratory musculature in combination with breathing and mobilization exercises for the trunk and thorax.

Rocking & Shaking

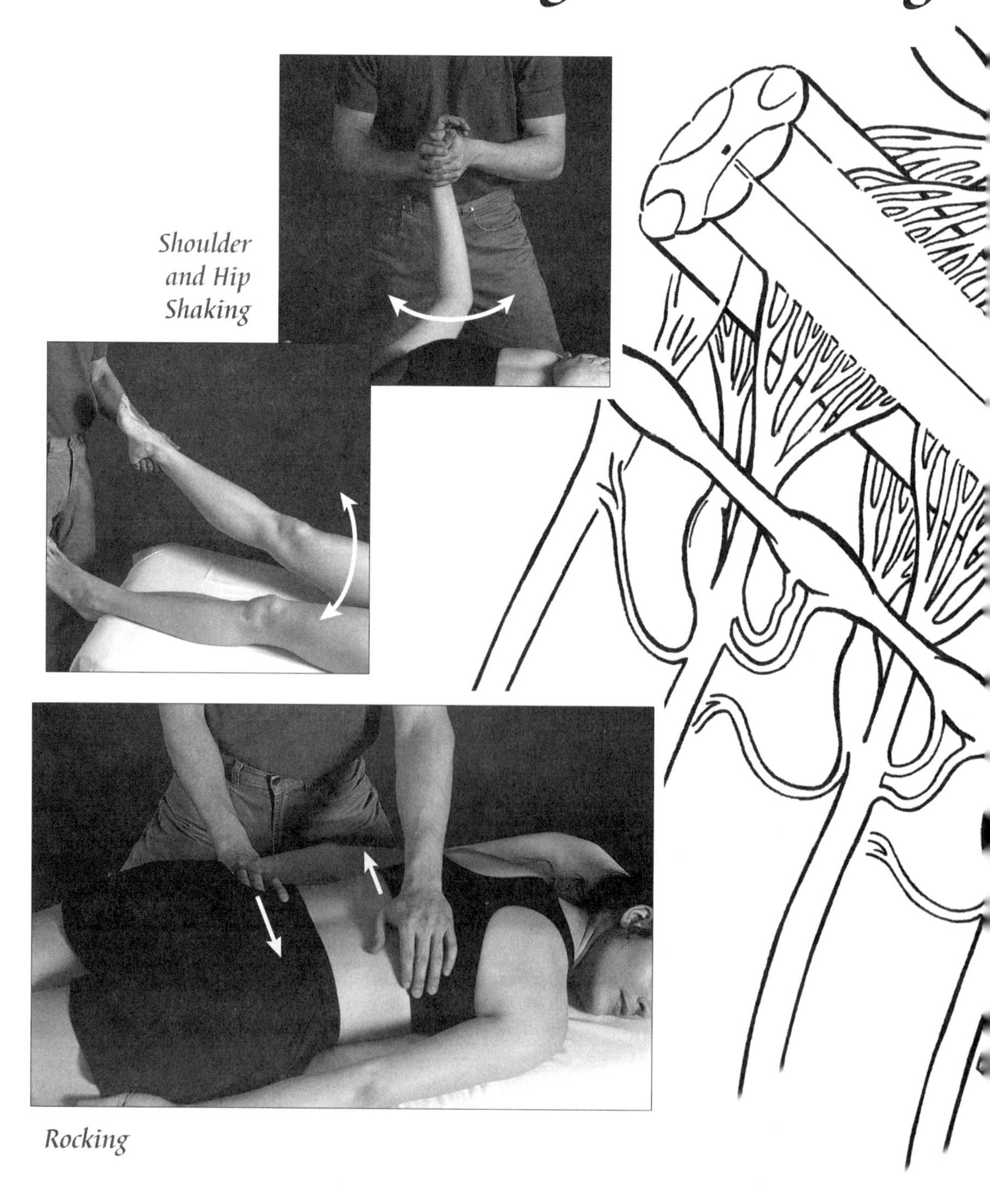

Shoulder and Hip Shaking

Rocking

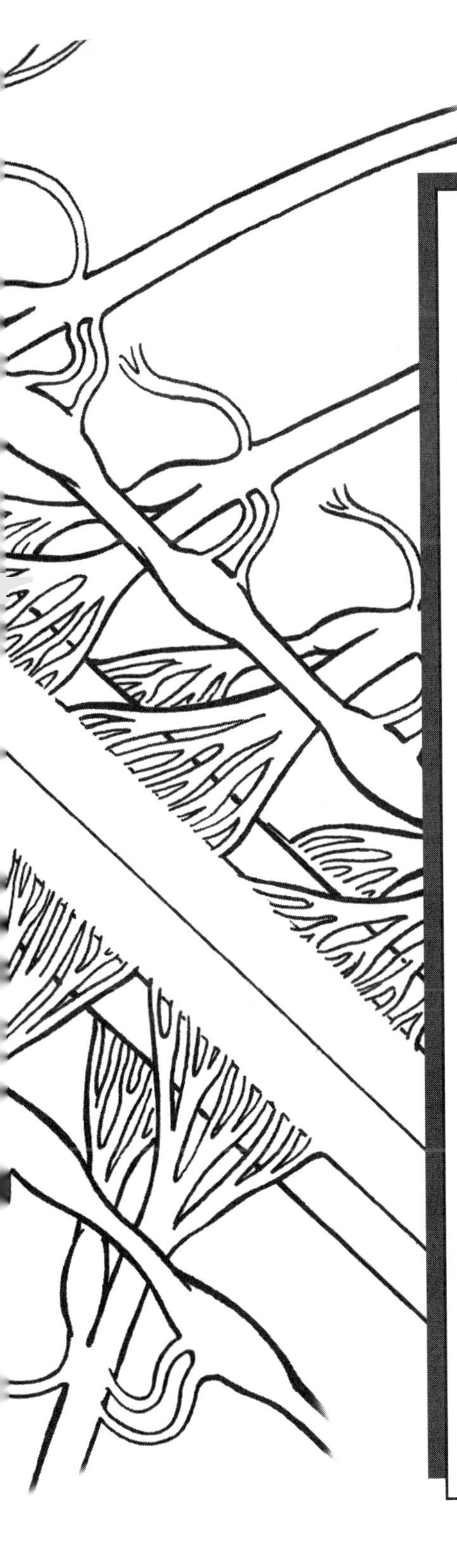

Rocking & Shaking

As a general rule, rocking gently moves the whole body while shaking is applied with varying degrees of rigor to body parts.

Customary Uses

Both

- Produce relaxing effects
- Increase proprioceptive input to reflexly decrease muscle tone
- Mobilize tight/stiff joints and related connective tissues
- Reduce psychologically based 'holding'
- Mobilize the thorax and increase ease of breathing
- Help prepare for more specific work

Rocking

- Soothing/nurturing effect for children and adults
- Sedative effect on pain and insomnia
- Reduces anxiety
- Facilitates ease of motion and awareness of resistant areas
- Produces a generalized decrease in postural tone
- Helps address muscle based low back conditions

Shaking

- Improves succussive action to rehabilitating or underused joints
- Can help align CT fibers during injury rehabilitation
- In sports massage, produces a mild rousing effect pre-event

Avoid (AV) or Adapt For (AD)

AV: Acute injuries to bones, soft tissues, nerves
AV: Joint instability/hypermobility
AV: Acute disc problems
AV: Spasticity
AV: Vertigo
AV: Recent local surgery
AD: Neuritis, chronic joint and soft tissue inflammatory conditions

7 Psychological Effects

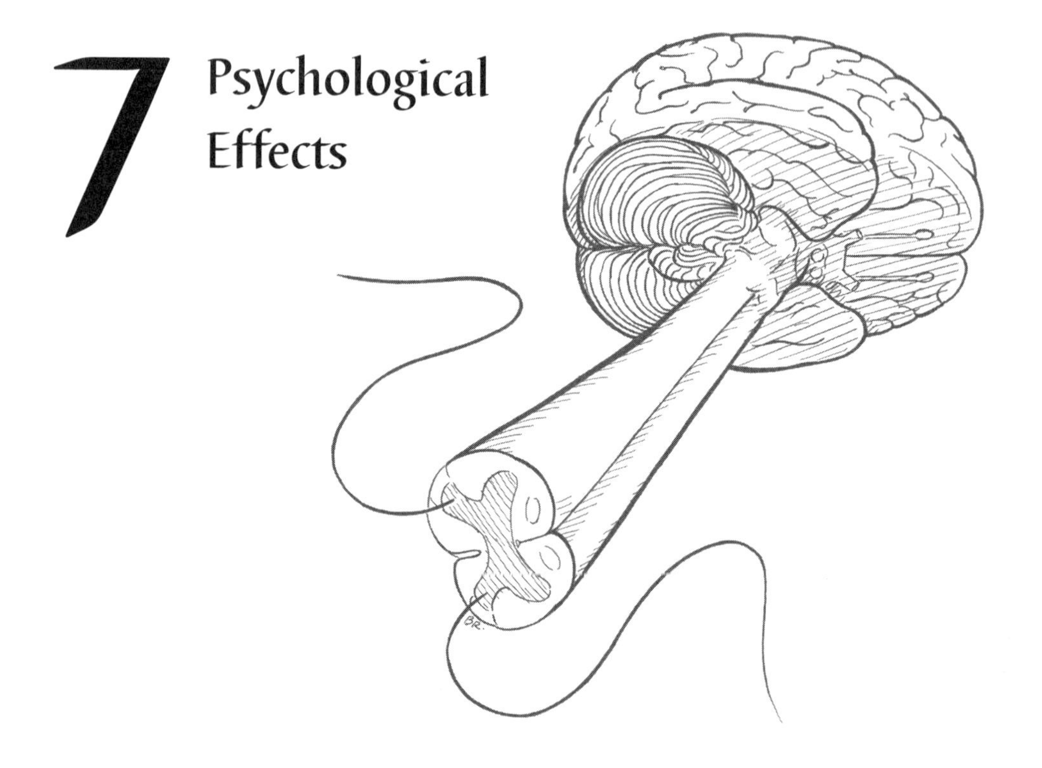

Massage is widely recognized as an effective tool for reducing anxiety, especially by those receiving regular treatment. Psychological effects appear to be the primary mechanism underlying the numerous non-specific benefits of massage identified in Chapter 1; reducing anxiety related to various causes and conditions is central to these effects. It is true, however, that massage therapy has not been sufficiently directed therapeutically for this purpose in patients who suffer from anxiety disorders. This potential application of massage therapy is beginning to receive more attention.

Fifteen minute chair massage in the workplace has been found to significantly reduce anxiety levels and systolic and diastolic blood pressures of recipients (Cady & Jones 1997; Shulman & Jones 1996). Field et al. (1996a) compared 15-minute chair massage to simply relaxing in the massage chair for 15 minutes and found that the massage group had reduced anxiety as measured by the State-Trait Anxiety Inventory (STAI) and the Profile of Mood States (POMS), and reduced stress hormones as indicated by salivary cortisol levels. In contrast to the relaxation subjects, decreased frontal alpha and beta power on EEG of the massage subjects suggested enhanced alertness. The massage group showed increased speed and accuracy on math computations post-intervention while the control group did not change.

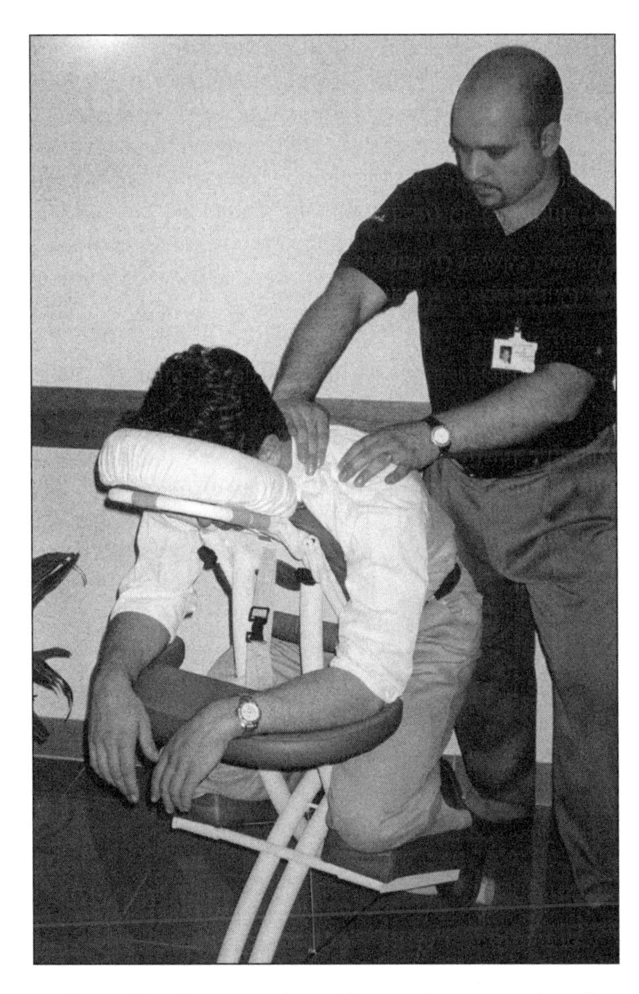

Meares (1980) discusses the use of massage as an adjunct to meditation in the treatment of cancer, as both serve to reduce anxiety. Longworth's (1982) study, described in Chapter 2, of the effects of slow stroke back massage on thirty-two normal female subjects leads this author to suggest that massage may be an effective intervention for individuals with high psycho-emotional or somatic arousal, and may be used effectively on cardiac and hypertensive patients as well. This conclusion has been supported by much subsequent research.

McKechnie et al. (1983) report the results of a pilot study involving five subjects with symptoms of chronic anxiety who had responded poorly to drug therapy. After receiving ten sessions of CTM, all subjects reported a diminution of symptoms, and three found they were able to discontinue their medication. Another pilot study was undertaken by Sims (1986) to examine the effects of gentle back massage on the perceived well-being of six female patients receiving radiotherapy for breast cancer. The subjects served as their own controls, reporting pre- and post-treatment levels of symptom distress and mood. Although the small sample size precluded statistically significant results, all six women reported less symptom distress, higher degrees of tranquility and vitality, and less tension and tiredness following the massage as compared to following the control intervention (a 10-minute rest period).

Fakouri and Jones (1987) undertook a study to assess the effectiveness of slow stroke massage in promoting general relaxation. The 18 subjects, ranging in age from 56 to 96 years (mean age 73.7), received massage each evening at bedtime on three consecutive nights. Rhythmic soothing stroking was done on the back for three minutes at a rate of about 60 strokes per minute. Heart rate, finger skin temperature, and systolic and diastolic blood pressure were recorded before, immediately after, and ten minutes after the massage. Heart rate and systolic BP were significantly reduced and skin temperature was significantly increased at both post-massage measurements on all three days. Diastolic BP did not reach a significant level of change until the third day, at which time it was reduced. These results strongly suggest that the slow stroke "back rub" promotes a relaxation response in elderly clients. In another study of the effects of back massage on elderly institutionalized patients, Fraser & Kerr (1993) found a statistically significant difference in the mean anxiety score between the back massage group as compared to the no-intervention group, and Richards (1998) reports that a 6-minute back massage is useful for promoting sleep in critically ill older men.

The Touch Research Institute of the University of Miami School of Medicine has conducted a number of interesting studies that evaluate the effect of massage on anxiety and depression. These studies have used the State-Trait Anxiety Inventory (STAI) or State Anxiety Inventory for Children (STAIC) and the Profile of Mood States (POMS) as psychological state measures as well as salivary and/or urinary cortisol levels as measures of stress hormone production.

1. Field et al. (1992) report that hospitalized child and adolescent psychiatric patients who received daily 30-minute massage for a five-day period were less anxious as measured by the STAIC and less depressed as measured by the POMS. Salivary cortisol levels were also reduced.

2. Ironson et al. (1996) report that daily massage of gay male subjects, some of whom were HIV+, for one month resulted in significantly decreased anxiety and increased relaxation (measured by STAI and POMS) and significantly decreased salivary and urinary cortisol levels. These changes were correlated with significant increases in several measures of immune function, including NK cell number, NK cell cytotoxicity, soluble CD8 and the cytotoxic subset of CD8 cells.

3. Field et al. (1996b) studied children whose scores on the PTSD Reaction Index suggested they were experiencing severe post-traumatic stress one month after hurricane Andrew. After receiving massage therapy for eight days they reported being happier and less anxious as measured by the Revised Children's Manifest Anxiety Scale (RCMAS) and STAIC, and also had lower salivary cortisol levels compared to children in a video attention group not receiving massage.

4. Fibromyalgia patients treated with massage reported fewer nights of difficult sleep, decreased anxiety as measured by the STAI, and less depression as measured by the POMS (Sunshine et al. 1996). Salivary cortisol levels were also reduced.
5. One month of daily 15-minute relaxation massages of children with juvenile rheumatoid arthritis resulted in decreased anxiety as measured by the STAIC, decreased salivary cortisol levels, and decreased pain as assessed by self-report, parent observation, and physician evaluation (Field et al. 1997a).
6. Massage therapy in adult burn patients also decreased STAI anxiety and cortisol levels, as well as decreased pain on the McGill Pain Questionnaire, Present Pain Intensity Scale, and Visual Analogue Scale (Field et al. 1998a).

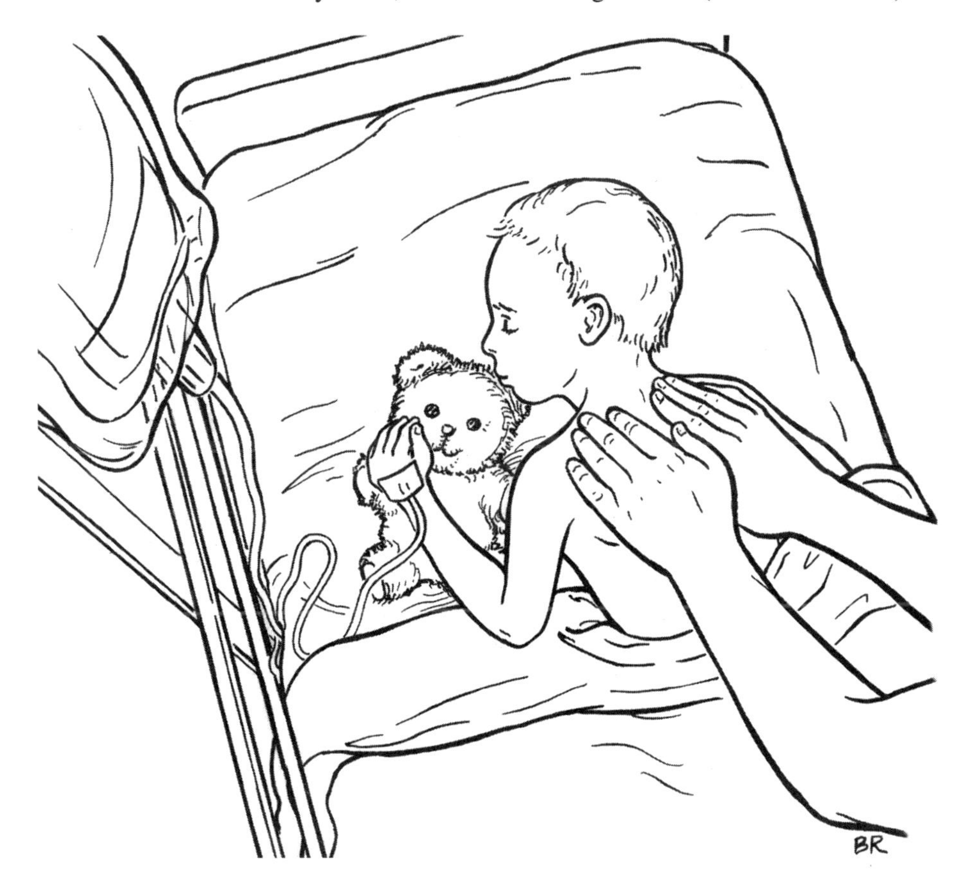

7. In a study of massage for children with asthma (Field et al. 1998b), decreased anxiety and cortisol levels as well as improved forced expiratory flow and other pulmonary function indicators were reported after treatment.
8. Bulimic adolescents who received 10 sessions of massage therapy over a five week period showed decreases in anxiety (STAI) and depression (POMS-D, self-report and behavior observation), associated with lower urinary cortisol levels and improved attitudes about eating disorder and body image (Field et al. 1997b).
9. Field et al. (1996c) report that depressed teenage mothers who received 10 30-minute massage therapy sessions over a 5-week period showed behavioral and stress hormone changes including lowered pulse readings and salivary and urinary cortisol levels, as well as decreases in anxious behavior.
10. In another study, (Field et al. 1997c) massaged mothers reported a decrease in depressed mood, anxiety, and pain, as well as having significantly shorter labors, shorter hospital stays, and less post-partum depression.
11. Field et al. (1998c) also report that massage therapy, but not relaxation therapy, of hyperactive children resulted in lower hyperactivity scores based on classroom behavior.

Applications in Pregnancy and Delivery

Massage therapy is an ideal nonpharmacological reducer of stress and anxiety for obstetric applications. Osborne-Sheets (1998) documents the following consequences of pre- and perinatal anxiety:

- increased maternal heart rate and blood pressure
- nausea and vomiting
- spontaneous abortion
- toxemia
- immune system dysfunction
- reduced uterine blood supply
- reduced fetal heart rate and blood oxygen saturation
- impaired fetal CNS development
- increased incidence of miscarriage, prematurity, labor and postpartum complications, low birth weight, and fetal distress

Osborne-Sheets further cites studies of the work of labor support professionals known as "doulas" who stroke, knead, hold and otherwise comfort women during labor, to the effect that such treatment results in 25% shorter labor times, 40% less need to use oxytocin as a labor stimulant, 30% reduction in use of pain medications and 60% reduction in epidural anesthesia, 40% less frequent need for forceps, and a 50% decreased incidence of caesarian sections (Klaus et al. 1993).

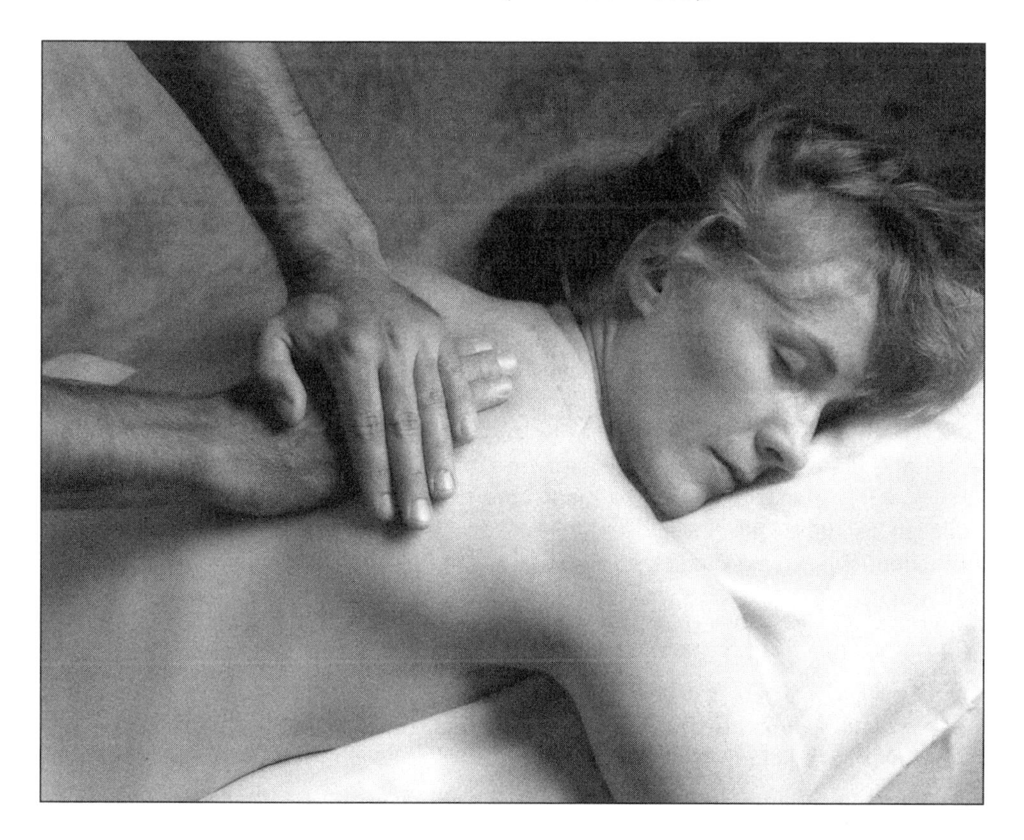

Indications for Massage Therapy

Massage therapy would appear to be indicated as a safe and effective inclusion in any therapeutic program focused on conditions characterized by anxiety/depression or individuals in life circumstances involving significant levels of anxiety. This broad set of indications would include a full spectrum of psychiatric, palliative, and hospice care scenarios and painful, stressful or frightening clinical procedures in both children and adults.

GLOSSARY OF MASSAGE THERAPY TERMS

Chair Massage:

Massage performed with the recipient in a sitting position, often utilizing a backless massage chair designed to provide support for the trunk and head while leaning forward.

Connective Tissue Massage (CTM):

A technique of applying strokes that produce a tangential pull on the skin to stimulate connective tissue reflex zones over the body surface. This technique is useful in loosening and relaxing tissues preparatory to therapeutic exercises following surgery or trauma, and is believed to have effects on the autonomic nervous system.

Deep Friction Massage:

A technique in which the hand remains in contact with the skin and the superficial tissues are moved with respect to the deeper tissues with the intention of disrupting collagenous adhesions. Deep friction massage is used to encourage optimal scar formation and to restore painless mobility of musculoskeletal structures, for example in tendinitis.

Transverse Friction Massage:

Deep friction massage in which the direction of movement is transverse to the orientation of the fibers in a muscle, tendon, ligament, or scar. Also known as cross-fiber friction.

Effleurage:

A core Swedish massage technique that utilizes smooth gliding pressures in a centripetal direction to promote lymph and venous drainage.

Hydrotherapy:

The systematic utilization of the thermal, mechanical, and chemical properties of water in hot, cold, or contrast temperature applications of various sizes, forms, and durations to produce beneficial therapeutic effects.

Joint Mobilization:

Passive traction and/or gliding movements applied to joint surfaces to restore or maintain joint play normally allowed by the capsule. The intention is to promote joint tissue nutrition and normal roll-slide joint mechanics. Controlled movement of a joint beyond the range that can be performed voluntarily is used where restriction exists due to tissue shortening and/or adhesion formation in the membranous structures associated with joints. Mobilizations performed by massage therapists do not include the high velocity, low amplitude thrust characteristic of chiropractic manipulations, nor are they used to increase the physiological range of healthy joints.

Manipulation:

The therapeutic application of external mechanical forces to body structures and tissues, or the forceful passive movement of a joint beyond its active limit of motion.

Manual Lymph Drainage (MLD):

Application of a series of gentle movements of light pressure, usually in a circular pattern, following the general distribution of lymph vessels draining a body region. The intention is to mimic the natural forces moving lymph fluids without disturbing the vascular circulation or triggering histamine release.

Manual Therapy:

Procedures by which all or parts of one or both hands directly contact the body to treat its soft tissues and articulations.

Massage:

The performance of a variety of manual techniques including stroking, kneading, manipulation, methodical pressure, friction, percussion, and vibration.

Massage Therapy:

The use of massage techniques, preceded by assessment and treatment planning, to address various conditions and patient (client) presentations, as well as to promote relaxation and enhanced well-being. Based on Swedish massage; however other techniques and modalities (for example, hydrotherapy) tend to be incorporated in relation to the therapist's ongoing education.

Myofascial Trigger Point Therapy:

The systematic location and release of active and latent myofascial trigger points (hyperirritable intramuscular foci) by means of focal deep pressure over the trigger point or a combination of vapocoolant spray and stretching. Trigger point therapy is used to decrease pain on active contraction of affected muscles. It is often applied prior to performing deep tissue massage, joint mobilizations, stretch, or remedial exercise.

Passive Movement:

Techniques by which the practitioner mobilizes body parts without active participation of the patient. Commonly involves repetitive movements of muscles and joints and associated structures over an increasing range in order to support tissue health, restore or improve mobility, reduce pain, and/or induce relaxation.

Petrissage:

A group of direct tissue techniques fundamental to Swedish massage that are characterized by specific kneading movements. Used primarily to address muscle and subcutaneous structures, they lift, squeeze and separate tissues.

Range of Motion (ROM):

Movements of joints to prevent loss of normal joint motion in all directions or to maximize restoration of range of movement following injury.

Active Range of Motion (AROM):

Movement, within the unrestricted range of motion that can be accomplished voluntarily, which is produced by active contraction of the muscles crossing a joint.

Active-Assisted Range of Motion (AAROM):

A type of active ROM in which assistance is provided by an outside force, either manually or mechanically, because the muscles require assistance to complete or sustain the motion.

Passive Range of Motion (PROM):

Movement, within the unrestricted range of motion for a segment, which is produced entirely by an external force without voluntary muscle contraction. Passive forced range of motion challenges restrictions and may be used to extend range of motion where limitations are present.

Remedial Exercise:

See Therapeutic Exercise.

Swedish Massage:

A system for inducing relaxation and treating the body's soft tissues through use of a series of techniques: palmar, digital, and knuckle movements, including effleurage and slow-stroke massage; kneading, rolling, and wringing manipulations (petrissage); frictions; vibration; percussion movements (tapotement); and rhythmic passive movements of joints and body parts.

Tapotement:

A group of percussive techniques used in massage therapy and physical therapy to create both mechanical and reflex effects, including respiratory passage clearance.

Therapeutic Exercise:

Corrective exercises utilized to enhance coordination, endurance, power, flexibility and range of motion. Also, exercise for the purpose of preventing adhesions, contractures, muscular atrophy, and loss of normal joint range of motion during recovery from injury or disease; or exercise for restoring compromised joint and muscle function, increasing muscular strength, and improving cardiovascular and pulmonary function. Therapeutic exercise includes therapist-assisted, therapist-supervised, and home exercise programs.

Therapeutic Stretch:

Therapeutic maneuvers intended to elongate soft tissue structures, especially when these are pathologically shortened, and thereby to increase function and range of motion.

Elastic Stretch:

Therapeutic stretch within the elastic limits of the connective tissue structures involved, and that does not result in mechanical alteration of tissue structure. Elastic stretch is believed to promote remodeling of connective tissue structures such as tendon and fascia to increase tissue extensibility.

Plastic Stretch:

Therapeutic stretch that exceeds the elastic limits of connective tissue, resulting in a mechanical alteration of tissue structures. Plastic stretch is intended to disrupt adhesions that may contribute to limited range of motion.

REFERENCES

Abrams SM. 2000. Attention-deficit/hyperactivity disordered children and adolescents benefit from massage therapy. *Dissertation Abstracts International - Section B: The Sciences and Engineering* 60: 5218.

Acolet D, Modi N, Giannakoulopoulos X, Bond C, Weg W, Clow A, Glover V. 1993. Changes in plasma cortisol and catecholamine concentrations in response to massage in preterm infants. *Arch Disease Child* 68:29-31.

Acosta AM, Chan RS, Jacobs J. 1998. Massage therapy for the treatment of painful peripheral neuropathy in HIV+ individuals. *Int Conf AIDS* 12:849.

Andrade CK, Clifford P. 2001. *Outcome-Based Massage*. Baltimore: Lippincott Williams & Wilkins.

Arkko PJ, Pakarinen AJ, Kari-Koskinen O. 1983. Effects of whole body massage on serum protein, electrolyte and hormone concentrations, enzyme activities and hematological parameters. *Int J Sports Med* 4:265-267.

Ashton J. 1984. Holistic Health. Six. In your hands. *Nurs Times* 80:54.

Askew LJ, Beckett VL, Kai Nan An, Chao EYS. 1983. Objective evaluation of hand function in scleroderma patients to assess effectiveness of physical therapy. *Br J Rheum* 22:224-232.

Bale P, James H. 1991. Massage, warm-down and rest as recuperative measures after short term intense exercise. *Physiother Sport* 13:4-7.

Barr JS, Taslitz N. 1970. The influence of back massage on autonomic functions. *Phys Ther* 50:1679-1691.

Basbaum A, Fields H. 1978. Endogenous pain control mechanisms: review and hypothesis. *Ann Neurol* 4:451-452.

Bauer W, Short CL, Bennett GA. 1933. The manner of removal of proteins from normal joints. *J Exper Med* 57:419.

Beeken JE, Parks D, Cory J, Montopoli G. 1998. The effectiveness of neuromuscular release massage therapy in five individuals with chronic obstructive lung disease. *Clin Nurs Res* 7:309-325.

Begin P, Grassino A. 1991. Inspiratory muscle dysfunction and chronic hypercapnea in chronic obstructive lung disease. *Amer Rev Respir Dis* 14:905-912.

Bierman W. 1955. Therapeutic use of cold. *JAMA* 157:1189-1192.

Billhult A, Dahlberg K. 2001. A meaningful relief from suffering. Experiences of massage in cancer care. *Cancer Nurs* 24:180-184.

Bodian M. 1969. Use of massage following lid surgery. *Eye Ear Nose Thr Mon* 48:542-547.

Boris M, Weindorf S, Lasinski B. 1997. Persistence of lymphedema reduction after noninvasive complex lymphedema therapy. *Oncology* 11:99-114.

Bowsher D. 1988. Modulation of nociceptive input. In: Wells PE, Frampton V, Bowsher D, ed. *Pain: Management and Control in Physiotherapy*. London: Heinemann Medical.

Breakey BM. 1982. An overlooked therapy you can use ad lib. *RN* 45:50-54.

Breslin EH. 1996. Respiratory muscle function in patients with chronic obstructive pulmonary disease. *Heart & Lung* 25:271-285.

Browse NL. 1986. The diagnosis and management of primary lymphedema. *J Vasc Surg* 3:181-184.

Bugaj R. 1975. The cooling, analgesic, and rewarming effects of ice massage on localized skin. *Phys Ther* 55(1):11-19.

Bumpus S. 1993. The effect of caring touch on the psychological well-being of selected residents of a long-term care facility. *S Carolina Nurse* 8:26-27.

Burke C, MacNish S, Saunders J, Gallini A, Warne I, Downing J. 1994. The development of a massage service for cancer patients. *Clin Oncol (Royal College of Radiologists)* 6:381-384.

Cady SH, Jones GE. 1997. Massage therapy as a workplace intervention for reduction of stress. *Percept Mot Skills* 84:157-158.

Campbell AH, O'Connell JM, Wilson F. 1975. The effect of chest physiotherapy upon FEV_1 in chronic bronchitis. *Med J Aust* 1:33-35.

Carrier EB. 1922. Studies on the physiology of capillaries. V. The reaction of the human skin capillaries to drugs and other stimuli. *Am J Physiol* 61:528-547.

Carter R, Coast JR. 1993. Respiratory muscle training in patients with chronic obstructive pulmonary disease. *J Cardiopulm Rehab* 13:117-125.

Castex A. 1891. Etude clinique et experimentale sur le massage. *Arch Gem Med* March: 278-302.

Chamberlain GJ. 1982. Cyriax's friction massage: a review. *J Orth Sports Phys Ther* 4:16-22.

Chang MY, Wang SY, Chen H. 2002. Effects of massage on pain and anxiety during labour: a randomized controlled trial in Taiwan. *J Adv Nurs* 38:68-73.

Cherkin DC, Eisenberg D, Sherman KJ, Barlow W, Kaptchuk TJ, Street J, Deyo RA. 2001. Randomized trial comparing traditional Chinese medical acupuncture, therapeutic massage, and self-care education for chronic low back pain. *Arch Intern Med* 161:1081-1088.

Cherkin DC, Sherman KJ, Deyo RA, Shekelle PG. 2003. A review of the evidence for the effectiveness, safety, and cost of acupuncture, massage therapy, and spinal manipulation for low back pain. *Ann Intern Med* 138:898-906.

Chopra SK, Laplin OV, Simmons DH, Robinson GDJr. 1977. Effects of hydration and physical therapy on tracheal transport velocity. *Am Rev Respir Dis* 115:1009-1014.

Chor H, Cleveland D, Davenport HA, Dolkart RE, Beard G. 1939. Atrophy and regeneration of the gastrocnemius-soleus muscles: Effects of physical therapy in monkey following section and suture of sciatic nerve. *JAMA* 113:1029-1033.

Chor H, Dolkart R. 1936. Study of simple disuse atrophy in the monkey. *Am J Physio* 117:4.

Cigales M, Field T, Lundy B, Cuadra A, Hart S. 1997. Massage enhances recovery from habituation in normal infants. *Infant Behav Dev* 20:29-34.

Clarke SW, Cochrane GM, Webber B. 1973. Cited in Chopra et al., 1977. Effects of sputum on pulmonary function. *Thorax* 28:262.

College of Massage Therapists of BC. 1997. *Curriculum Standard.* Vancouver: College of Massage Therapists of British Columbia.

Corbett M. 1972. The use and abuse of massage and exercise. *Practitioner* 208:136-139.

Cotton LT, Roberts VC. 1977. The prevention of deep vein thrombosis, with particular reference to mechanical methods of prevention. *Surgery* 81:228-235.

Crosman LJ, Chateauvert SR, Weisberg J. 1984. The effects of massage to the hamstring muscle group on range of motion. *JOSPT* 6(3):168-172.

Culpepper-Richards K, 1998. Effect of a back massage and relaxation intervention on sleep in critically ill patients. *Am J Crit Care* 7:288-299.

Curtis M. 1994. The use of massage in restoring cardiac rhythm. *Nurs Times* 90:36-37

Cuthbertson DP. 1933. Effect of massage on metabolism. A survey. *Glasgow Med J* (New 7th Series) 2:200-213.

Cyriax JH. 1960. Clinical applications of massage. In: Licht S. ed. *Massage, Manipulation and Traction.* Huntington, NY: Robert E Krieger Publishing Co, 1976. (Reprint of Licht E. New Haven, 1960, which was issued as Vol 5 of *Physical Medicine Library*).

Cyriax J. 1977. Deep Massage. *Physiotherapy* 63:60-61.

Cyriax J. 1984a. Theory and practice of massage. *Textbook of Orthopaedic Medicine*. Vol 2, *Treatment by Manipulation, Massage and Injection*. 11th ed. Toronto: Bailliere Tindall.

Cyriax J. 1984b. Passive movement. *Textbook of Orthopaedic Medicine*. Vol 2, *Treatment by Manipulation, Massage and Injection*. 11th ed. Toronto: Bailliere Tindall.

Cyriax J. 1984c. Indications for and against deep friction. *Textbook of Orthopaedic Medicine*. Vol 2, *Treatment by Manipulation, Massage and Injection*. 11th ed. Toronto: Bailliere Tindall.

Dallimore K, Jenkins S, Tucker B. 1998. Respiratory and cardiovascular responses to manual chest percussion in normal subjects. *Aust J Physiother* 44:267-274.

Danneskiold-Samsoe B, Christianson E, Lund B, Anderson RB. 1982. Regional muscle tension and pain (fibrositis). Effect of massage on myoglobin in plasma. *Scand J Rehab Med* 15:17-20.

Danneskiold-Samsoe B, Christianson E, Anderson RB 1986. Myofascial pain and the role of myoglobin. *Scand J Rheum* (Stockholm) 15:174-178.

Dawson P, Kontos P. 1998. Back massage can reduce anxiety of elderly residents in long-term care institutions. *Perspectives* 22:27.

Day JA, Mason RR, Chesrown SE. 1987. Effect of massage on serum level of beta-endorphin and beta-lipotropin in healthy adults. *Phys Ther* 67:926-930.

de Bruijn R. 1984. Deep transverse friction: its analgesic effect. *Int J Sports Med* 5(suppl):35-36.

Delaney JP, Leong KS, Watkins A, Brodie D. 2002. The short-term effects of myofascial trigger point massage therapy on cardiac autonomic tone in healthy subjects. *J Adv Nurs* 37:364-371.

Denny-Brown D, Adams RD, Brenner C, Doherty MM. 1945. The pathology of injury to nerve induced by cold. *J Neuropath Exp Neurol* 4:305-323.

Diego MA, Field T, Hernandez-Reif M, Hart S, Brucker B, Field T, Burman I. 2002. Spinal cord patients benefit from massage therapy. *Int J Neurosci* 112:133-142.

Diego MA, Hernandez-Reif M, Field T, Friedman L, Shaw K. 2001. HIV adolescents show improved immune function following massage therapy. *Int J Neurosci* 106:35-45.

Doering TJ, Fieguth HG, Steuernagel B, Brix J, Konitzer M, Schneider B, Fischer GC. 1999. External stimuli in the form of vibratory massage after heart or lung transplantation. *Am J Phys Med Rehab* 78:108-110.

Dossetor DR, Couryer S, Nicol AR. 1991. Massage for very severe self-injurious behaviour in a girl with Cornelia de Lange syndrome. *Dev Med Child Neurol* 33:636-640.

Drinker CK. 1939. The formation and movements of lymph. *Am Heart J* 18:389.

Drinker CK, Yoffey JM. 1941. *Lymphatics, Lymph, and Lymphoid Tissue: Their Physiological and Clinical Significance*. Cambridge: Harvard University Press.

Ebner M. 1975. *Connective Tissue Massage: Theory and Therapeutic Application*. 2nd ed. Edinburgh and London: E & S Livingston Ltd.

Edgecombe W, Bain W. 1899. The effect of baths, massage and exercise on the blood pressure. *Lancet* 1:1552.

Einfeldt H, Henkel M, Schmidt-Auffurth T, Lange G. 1986. Therapeutische und palliative lymphdrainage zur odentherapie im gesichts-und halsbereich. *HNQ* 34:365-367.

Eisenberg D, Davis R, Ettner S, Appel S, Wilkey S, Van Rompay M, Kessler RC. 1998. Trends in Alternative Medicine Use in the United States, 1990-1997, *JAMA* 280:1569-1575.

Elkins EC, Herrick JF, Grindlay JH, Mann FC, De Forest RE. 1953. Effect of various procedures on the flow of lymph. *Arch Phys Med* 34:31-39.

Ellison M, Goerhrs C, Hall L, et al. 1992. Effect of retrograde massage on muscle soreness and performance. [abstract] *Phys Ther* 72:100.

Ernst E. 1998. Does post-exercise massage treatment reduce delayed onset muscle soreness? A systematic review. *Br J Sports Med* 32:212-214.

Ernst E. 1999. Massage therapy for low back pain: a systematic review. *J Pain Sympt Mgt* 17:65-69.

Ernst E. 2003. The safety of massage therapy. *Rheumatology* 42:1101-1106.

Ernst E. 2003. Manual therapies for pain control: chiropractic and massage. *Clin J Pain* 20:8-12.

Ernst E, Matrai A, Magyarosy I, Liebermeister RGA, Eck M, Breu MC. 1987. Massages cause changes in blood fluidity. *Physiotherapy* 73:43-45.

Escalona A, Field T, Singer-Strunk R, Cullen C, Hartshorn K. 2001. Improvements in the behavior of children with autism. *J Autism Dev Disord* 31:513-516.

Fakouri C, Jones P. 1987. Relaxation Rx: slow stroke back rub. *J Gerontol Nurs* 13:32-35.

Farr T, Nottle C, Nosaka K, Sacco P. 2002. The effects of massage on delayed onset muscle soreness and muscle function following downhill walking. *Sci Med Sport* 5:297-306.

Fassbender HG, Wegner K. 1973. Cited in Danneskiold-Samsoe et al., 1986. Morphologie und Pathogenese des Weichteilrheumatismus. *Z Rheumaforsch* 32:355-374.

Ferber SG, Kuint J, Weller A, Feldman R, Dollberg S, Arbel E, Kohelet D. 2002. Massage therapy by mothers and trained professionals enhances weight gain in preterm infants. *Early Human Dev* 67:37-45

Ferrell-Torry AT, Glick OJ. 1993. The use of therapeutic massage as a nursing intervention to modify anxiety and the perception of cancer pain. *Cancer Nurs* 16:93-101.

Field T. 1987. Alleviating stress in NICU neonates. *JAOA* 87: 646-650.

Field T. 1990. Alleviating stress in newborn infants in the intensive care unit. *Perinatology* 17:1-9.

Field T. 1992. Interventions in early infancy. Special Section: Australian Regional Meeting: Attachment and the relationship between the infant and caregivers. *Infant Ment Health J* 13:329-336.

Field T. 1995. Massage therapy for infants and children. [Review]. *J Dev Behav Ped* 16:105-111.

Field T. 1998. Massage therapy effects. *Amer Psychologist* 53:1270-1281.

Field T, Hernandez-Reif M. 2001. Sleep problems in infants decrease following massage therapy. *Early Child Dev Care* 168:95-104.

Field T, Schanberg SM, Scafidi F, Bauer CR, Vega-Lahr N, Garcia R, Nystrom J, Kuhn CM. 1986. Tactile/kinesthetic stimulation effects on preterm neonates. *Pediatrics* 77:654-658.

Field T, Morrow C, Valdeon C, Larson S, Kuhn C, Schanberg S. 1992. Massage reduces anxiety in child and adolescent psychiatric patients. *J Am Acad Child Adolesc Psychiatry* 31(1):125-128.

Field T, Ironson G, Scafidi F, Nawrocki T, Goncalves A, Pickens J, Fox N, Schanberg S, Kuhn C. 1996a. Massage therapy reduces anxiety and enhances EEG pattern of alertness and math computations. *Int J Neurosci* 86:197-205.

Field T, Seligman S, Scafidi F, Schanberg S. 1996b. Alleviating post-traumatic stress in children following hurricane Andrew. *J App Dev Psychol* 17(1):37-50.

Field T, Grizzle N, Scafidi F, Schanberg S. 1996c. Massage and relaxation therapies' effects on depressed adolescent mothers. *Adolescence* 31:903-911.

Field T, Grizzle N, Scafidi F, Abrams S, Richardson S. 1996d. Massage therapy for infants of depressed mothers. *Infant Behav Dev* 19:109-114.

Field T, Kilmer T, Hernandez-Reif M, Burman I. 1996e. Preschool children's sleep and wake behavior: effects of massage therapy. *Early Child Dev Care* 120:39-44.

Field T, Hernandez-Reif M, Seligman S, Krasnegor J, Sunshine W, Rivas-Chacon R, Schanberg S. 1997a. Juvenile rheumatoid arthritis: benefits from massage therapy. *J Pediatr Psychol* 22:607-617.

Field T, Schanberg S, Kuhn C, Fierro K, Henteleff T, Mueller C, Yando R, Burman I. 1997b. Bulimic adolescents benefit from massage therapy. *Adolescence* 131:555-563.

Field T, Hernandez-Reif M, Taylor S, Quintano O, Burman I. 1997c. Labor pain is reduced by massage therapy. *J Psychosom Obstet Gynaecol* 18:286-291.

Field T, Hernandez-Reif M, Hart S, Quintino O, Drose L, Field T, Kuhn C, Schanberg S. 1997d. Sexual abuse effects are lessened by massage therapy. *J Bodyw Mov Ther* 1:65-69.

Field T, Hernandez-Reif M, LaGreca A, Shaw K, Schanberg S, Kuhn C. 1997e. Massage therapy lowers blood glucose levels in children with diabetes mellitus. *Diab Spectrum* 10:237-239.

Field T, Sunshine W, Hernandez-Reif M, Quintino O, Schanberg S, Kuhn C, Burman I. 1997f. Chronic fatigue syndrome: massage therapy effects on depression and somatic symptoms in chronic fatigue syndrome. *J Chron Fatig Syndr* 3:43-51.

Field T, Quintino O, Henteleff T, Wells-Keife L, Delvecchio-Feinberg G. 1997g. Job stress reduction therapies. *Alt Ther Health Med* 3:54-56.

Field T, Lasko D, Mundy P, Henteleff T, Talpins S, Dowling M. 1997h. Autistic children's attentiveness and responsivity improve after touch therapy. *J Autism Dev Disord* 27:333-338.

Field T, Peck M, Krugman S, Tuchel T, Schanberg S, Kuhn C, Burman I. 1998a. Burn injuries benefit from massage therapy. *J Burn Care Rehab* 19:241-244.

Field T, Henteleff T, Hernandez-Reif M, Martinez E, Mavunda K, Kuhn C, Schanberg S. 1998b. Children with asthma have improved pulmonary functions after massage therapy. *J Pediatr* 132:854-858.

Field TM, Quintano O, Hernandez-Reif M, Koslovsky G. 1998c. Adolescents with attention deficit disorder benefit from massage therapy. *Adolescence* 33:103-108.

Field T, Hernandez-Reif M, Hart S, Theakston H, Schanberg S, Kuhn C, Burman I. 1999. Pregnant women benefit from massage therapy. *J Psychosom Obstet Gynaecol* 20:31-38.

Field T, Peck M, Hernandez-Reif M, Krugman S, Burman I, Ozment-Schenck L. 2000. Postburn itching, pain, and psychological symptoms are reduced with massage therapy. *J Burn Care Rehab* 21:189-93.

Field T, Cullen C, Diego M, Hernandez-Reif M, Sprinz P, Beebe K, Kissel B, Bango-Sanchez V. 2001. Leukemia immune changes following massage therapy. *J Bodyw Mov Ther* 5:271-274.

Flowers KR. 1988. String wrapping versus massage for reducing digital volume. *Phys Ther* 68:57-59.

Foldi M. 1978. Anatomical and physiological basis for physical therapy of lymphedema. *Experientia* 33(suppl):15-18.

Fraser J, Kerr JR. 1993. Psychophysiological effects of back massage on elderly institutionalized patients. *J Adv Nurs* 18:238-245.

Frazer FW. 1978. Persistent post-sympathetic pain treated by connective tissue massage. *Physiotherapy* 64:211-212.

Furlan AD, Brosseau L, Imamura M, Irvin E. 2000. Massage for low back pain. *Cochr Database Syst Rev*(2):CD001929.

Gibson A. 1988. Back injuries: A hands-on approach. *AAOHN Journal* 36:218-223.

Gifford J, Gifford L. 1988. Chapter 14. Connective tissue massage. In: Wells PE, Frampton V, Bowsher D, ed. *Pain: Management and Control in Physiotherapy*. London: Heinemann Medical.

Goats GC. 1990. Interferential current therapy. *Br J Sports Med* 24:87-92.

Goats GC. 1994. Massage - the scientific basis of an ancient art: Part 2. Physiological and therapeutic effects. *Br J Sports Med* 28(3):153.

Goats GC, Keir K. 1991. Connective tissue massage. *Br J Sports Med* 25:131-133.

Goldberg J, Sullivan SJ, Seaborne DE. 1992. The effect of two intensities of massage on H-reflex amplitude. *Phys Ther* 72(6):449-457.

Goldberg J, Seaborne DE, Sullivan SJ, Leduc BE. 1994. The effect of therapeutic massage on H-reflex amplitude in persons with a spinal cord injury. *Phys Ther* 74(8):728-737.

Graham D. 1913. *Massage, Manual Treatment, Remedial Movements, History, Mode of Application and Effects: Indications and Contra-indications*. Philadelphia: J.P. Lippincott.

Grant AE. 1964. Massage with ice (cryokinetics) in the treatment of painful conditions of the musculoskeletal system. *Arch Phys Med* 45:233-238.

Grealish L, Lomasney A, Whiteman B. 2000. Foot massage. A nursing intervention to modify the distressing symptoms of pain and nausea in patients hospitalized with cancer. *Cancer Nurs* 23:237-43.

Gray B (1987). Management of limb oedema in advanced cancer. *Nurs Times* 83:39-41

Grieve GP. 1981. *Common Vertebral Joint Problems*. Edinburgh: Churchill Livingstone.

Hammer WI. 1993. The use of transverse friction massage in the management of chronic bursitis of the hip and shoulder. *J Manipulative Physio Ther* 16(2):107-111.

Hammon WE, McCaffree DR, Cucchiara AJ. 1993. A comparison of manual to mechanical chest percussion for clearance of alveolar material in patients with pulmonary alveolar proteinosis (phospholipidosis). *Chest* 103:1409-1412.

Hansen TI, Kristensen JH. 1973. Effect of massage, shortwave diathermy and ultrasound upon 133Xe disappearance rate from muscle and subcutaneous tissue in the human calf. *Scand J Rehab Med* 5:179-182.

Harris J. 1986. Managing massage in the fitness center. *Fitness Mgt* Nov/Dec: 8-12.

Hart S, Field T, Hernandez-Reif M, Lundy B. 1998. Preschoolers' cognitive performance improves following massage. *Early Child Dev Care* 143:59-64.

Hart S, Field T, Hernandez-Reif M, Nearing G, Shaw S, Schanberg S, Kuhn C. 2001. Anorexia symptoms are reduced by massage therapy. *Eating Disord* 9:289-299.

Hayden C.A. 1964. Cryokinetics in an early treatment program. *Phys Ther* 44:990-993.

Heipertz W. 1963. *Fortschr der Mediz* 81:454.

Heipertz W. 1965. *Archiv orthop u Unfall Chir* 57:214.

Hemmings B, Smith M, Graydon J, Dyson R. 2000. Effects of massage on physiological restoration, perceived recovery, and repeated sports performance. *Br J Sports Med* 34:109-115.

Hemphill L, Kemp J. 2000. Implementing a therapeutic massage program in a tertiary and ambulatory care VA setting: the healing power of touch. *Nurs Clin N Amer* 35:489-497.

Hernandez-Reif M, Field T, Dieter J, Swerdlow U, Diego M. 1998a. Migraine headaches were reduced by massage therapy. *Int J Neurosci* 96:1-11.

Hernandez-Reif M, Field T, Largie S, Hart S, Redzepi M, Nierenberg B, Peck M. 2001a. Childrens' distress during burn treatment is reduced by massage therapy. *J Burn Care Rehab* 22:191-195.

Hernandez-Reif M, Field T, Krasnegor J, Martinez E, Schwartzman M, Mavunda K. 1999. Children with cystic fibrosis benefit from massage therapy. *J Ped Psychol* 24:175-181.

Hernandez-Reif M, Field T, Krasnegor J, Theakston H. 2001b. Lower back pain is reduced and range of motion increased after massage therapy. *Int J Neurosci* 106:131-145.

Hernandez-Reif M, Field T, Krasnegor J, Theakston H, Burman I. 2000a. Chronic lower back pain is reduced and range of motion improved with massage therapy. *Int J Neurosci* 99:1-15.

Hernandez-Reif M, Field T, Theakston H. 1998b. Multiple sclerosis patients benefit from massage therapy. *J Bodyw Mov Ther* 2:168-174.

Hernandez-Reif M, Martinez A, Field T, Quintero O, Hart S. 2000b. Premenstrual syndrome symptoms are relieved by massage therapy. *J Psychosom Obstet Gynecol* 21:9-15.

Hilbert JE, Sforzo GA, Swenson T. 2003. The effects of massage on delayed onset muscle soreness. *Br J Sports Med* 37:72-75.

Hilliard D. 1995. Massage for the seriously mentally ill. *J Psychosoc Nurs Ment Health Serv* 33:29-30.

Howard SB, Krishnagiri S. 2001. The use of manual edema mobilization for the reduction of persistent edema in the upper limb. *J Hand Ther* 14:291-301.

Huddleston OL, Austin E, Moore RW, Cailliet R, Rubin D. 1952. Anterior poliomyelitis: physical treatment in Southern California. *Brit J Phys Med* 15:75.

Hutzschenreuter P, Wittlinger H, Wittlinger G, Kurz I. 1991. Post-mastectomy arm lymphedema: treated by manual lymph drainage and compression bandage therapy. *PMR* 1:166-170.

Hutzschenreuter P, Wittlinger G, Kurz I. 1992. Das sekundare postmastektomie-armlymphodem nach manueller lymphdrainage-behandlungen und kompressionstherapie. *Schriftenreihe Manuelle Lymphdrainage nach Dr. Vodder* 3:41-43.

Hutzschenreuter P, Herpertz U. 1993. Primary and secondary lymphedema in children treated with manual lymph drainage and compression therapy. *Lymphology* 4:51-57.

Inagaki J, Yoneda J, Ito M, Nogaki H. 2002. Psychophysiological effect of massage and shiatsu while in the prone position with the face down. *Nurs Health Sci* 4:A5-6.

Ironson G, Field T, Scafidi F, Hashimoto M, Kumar M, Kumar A, Price A, Gonclaves A, Burman I, Tetenman C, Patarca R, Fletcher MA. 1996. Massage therapy is associated with enhancement of the immune system's cytotoxic capacity. *Int J Neurosci* 84:205-217.

Irwin S, Tecklin JS, eds. 1995. *Cardiopulmonary Physical Therapy*. 3rd ed. St. Louis: Mosby

Jacobs M. 1960. Massage for the relief of pain: anatomical and physiological considerations. *Phys Ther Rev* 40:93-98.

Jones N, Field T. 1999. Right frontal EEG asymmetry is attenuated by massage and music therapy. *Adolescence* 34:529-534.

Kaada B, Torsteinbo O. 1989. Increase of plasma beta-endorphins in connective tissue massage. *Gen Pharmacol* 20:487-489.

Kaaja R, Tiula E. 1989. Manual lymph drainage in nephrotic syndrome during pregnancy. *Lancet* Oct. 21:990.

Kantrowitz FG, Farrar DJ, Locke SE. 1995. Chronic fatigue syndrome. 2: Treatment and future research. *Behav Med* 21:17-24.

Kisner CD, Taslitz N. 1968. Connective tissue massage: influence of the introductory treatment on autonomic functions. *Phys Ther* 48:107-119.

Klaus MH, Kennell JH, Klaus PH. 1993. *Mothering the Mother: How a Doula Can Help You Have a Shorter, Easier, and Healthier Birth.* p.51. Reading, MA. Addison-Wesley.

Knight MTN, Dawson R. 1976. Effect of intermittent compression of the arms on deep vein thrombosis in the legs. *Lancet* ii:1265-1267.

Ko DS, Lerner R, Klose G, Cosimi AB. 1998. Effective treatment of lymphedema of the extremities. *Arch Surg* 133:452-458.

Korr IM. 1975. Proprioceptors and somatic dysfunction. *JAOA* 74:638-650.

Kouri JP. 1992. Fibromyalgie - krankheitsbild und therapeutische ergebnisse. *Schriftenreihe Manuelle Lymphdrainage nach Dr. Vodder* 3:133-136.

Kriederman B, Myloyde T, Bernas M, Lee-Donaldson L, Preciado S, Lynch M, Stea B, Summers P, Witte C, Witte M. 2002. Limb volume reduction after physical treatment by compression and/or massage in a rodent model of peripheral lymphedema. *Lymphology* 35:23-27.

Krilov VN, Talishev FM, Burovikh AN. 1985. The use of restorative massage in the training of high level basketball players. *Sov Sports Rev* 20:7-9.

Kurz W, Wittlinger G, Litmanovitch YI, Romanoff H, Pfeifer Y, Tal E, Sulman FG. 1978. Effect of manual lymph drainage massage on urinary excretion of neurohormones and minerals in chronic lymphedema. *Angiology* 29:764-772.

Ladd MP, Kottke FJ, Blanchard RS. 1952. Studies of the effect of massage on the flow of lymph from the foreleg of the dog. *Arch Phys Med* 33:604-612.

Lerner R. 1998. What's new in lymphedema therapy in America? *Int J Angiol* 7:191-196.

Leroy MR. 1941. La vie du tissu conjunctif et sa defense par le massage. *Revue Medicale de Paris* 58:212.

Li ZM. 1984. 235 cases of frozen shoulder treated by manipulation and massage. *J Tradit Chin Med* 4:213-215.

Linde B. 1986. Dissociation of insulin absorption and blood flow during massage of a subcutaneous injection site. *Diab Care* 6:570-574.

Little L, Porche DJ. 1998. Manual lymph drainage (MLD). *J Assoc Nurses AIDS Care* 9:78-81.

Longworth JCD. 1982. Psychophysiological effects of slow stroke back massage in normotensive females. *Adv Nurs Sci* 4:44-61.

Lund I, Yu LC, Uvnas-Moberg K, Wang J, Yu C, Kurosawa M, Agren G, Rosen A, Lekman M, Lundberg T. 2002. Repeated massage-like stimulation induces long-term effects on nociception: contribution of oxytocinergic mechanisms. *Eur J Neurosci* 16:330-338.

MacGregor M. 1971. Manual treatment at the knee. *Physiotherapy* 57:207-211.

Mainusch H. 1992. Sklerodermie erfolgreich behandeln; manuelle lymphdrainage - ein therapiekozept. *Physikalisch Therapie* June:432-435.

Marshall CM. 1971. The use of ice-cube massage for the relief of chronic pain following herpes opthalmicus. *Physiotherapy* 57:374.

Matheson DW, Edelson R, Hiatrides D, Newkirk J, Twinem K, Thurston S. 1976. Relaxation measured by EMG as a function of vibrotactile stimulation. *Biofeedback Self Regul* 1:285-292.

Matusezewski W. 1985. Rehabilitative regeneration in sport. *SPORTS* Jan: Part 1; June: Part 2.

McKechnie AA, Wilson P, Watson N, Scott D. 1983. Anxiety states: a preliminary report on the value of connective tissue massage. *J Psychosom Res* 27:125-129.

McKinney LA. 1989. Early mobilization and outcome in acute sprains of the neck. *BMJ* 299:1006-1008.

Mealy K, Brennan H, Fenelson GCC. 1986. Early mobilization of acute whiplash injuries. *BMJ* 292:656-657.

Meares A. 1980. Massage as an adjunct to meditation in the psychological treatment of cancer. *Aust J Physiother* 26:25-26.

Meek SS. 1993. Effects of slow stroke back massage on relaxation in hospice clients. *J Nurs Schol* 25:17-21.

Melrose DG, Knight MTN, Simandl E. 1979. The stripping of varicose veins: a clinical trial of intermittent compression dressings. *Br J Surg* 66:53-55.

Melzack R, Bentley KC. 1983. Relief of dental pain by ice massage of either hand or the contralateral arm. *J Can Dent Assoc* 49:257-260.

Melzack R, Jeans ME, Stratford JG, Monks RC. 1980a. Ice massage and transcutaneous electrical stimulation: comparison of treatment for low back pain. *Pain* 9:209-217.

Melzack R, Guite S, Gonshor A. 1980b. Relief of dental pain by ice massage of the hand. *Can Med Assoc J* 122:189-191.

Melzack R, Wall PD. 1965. Pain mechanisms: a new theory. *Science* 150:971-979.

Mennel, J. 1945. *Physical Treatment by Movement, Manipulation and Massage*. 5th ed. Philadelphia: Blakiston Co.

Mobily PR, Herr KA, Nicholson AC. 1994. Validation of cutaneous stimulation interventions for pain management. *Int J Nurs Stud* 31:533-544.

Morelli M, Seaborne DE, Sullivan SJ. 1990. Changes in H-reflex amplitude during massage of triceps surae in healthy subjects. *JOSPT* 12(2):55-59.

Morgan RG, Casley-Smith JR, Mason MR. 1992. Complex physical therapy for the lymphoedematous arm. *J Hand Surg - British Vol* 17:437-441.

Murphy AJ. 1959. The physiological effects of cold application. Presented at the Annual Conference of the American Physical Therapy Association, Minneapolis, June, 1959.

Newman S. 1986a. Canada's case for sports massage. *Coaching Rev* May/June:20-25.

Newman S. 1986b. Canadian athletes and massage. *Coaching Rev* May/June:16-20.

Nixon M, Teschendorff J, Finney J, Karnilowicz W. 1997. Expanding the nursing repertoire: the effect of massage on post-operative pain. *Aust J Adv Nurs* 14:21-26.

Nordschow M, Bierman W. 1962. Influence of manual massage on muscle relaxation. *Phys Ther* 42:653-657.

Offenbacher M, Stucki G. 2000. Physical therapy in the treatment of fibromyalgia. *Scand J Rheum - Suppl* 113:78-85.

Onozawa K, Glover V, Adams D, Modi N, Kumar RC. 2001. Infant massage improves mother-infant interaction for mothers with postnatal depression. *J Aff Disord* 63:1-3.

Osborne-Sheets C. 1998. *Pre- and Perinatal Massage Therapy*. p.3. San Diego, CA. Body Therapy Associates.

Paikov VB. 1985. Means of restoration in training of speed skaters. *Sov Sports Rev* 20:7-12

Pemberton, R. 1950. Physiology of massage, in *A.M.A. Handbook of Physical Medicine and Rehabilitation*. Toronto: Blakiston Co.

Pflug JJ. 1974. Intermittent compression: a new principle in treatment of wounds. *Lancet* ii:355-366.

Pflug JJ. 1975. Intermittent compression in the management of swollen legs in general practice. *Practitioner* 215:69-76.

Pham QT, Peslin R, Puchelle E, Salmon D, Caraux G, Benis AM. 1973. Cited in Chopra et al., 1977. Respiratory function and the rheological status of bronchial secretions collected by spontaneous expectoration and after physiotherapy. *Bull Physiopathol Respir (Nancy)* 9:292.

Pope MH, Phillips RB, Haugh LD, Hsieh CY, MacDonald L, Haldeman S. 1994. A prospective randomized three-week trial of spinal manipulation, trans-cutaneous muscle stimulation, massage and corset in the treatment of subacute low back pain. *Spine* 19:2571-2577.

Preyde M. 2000. Effectiveness of massage therapy for subacute low-back pain: a randomized controlled trial. *CMAJ* 162(13):1815-1820.

Puusjarvi K, Airaksinen O, Pontinen PJ. 1990. The effects of massage in patients with chronic tension headache. *Acupuncture & Electro-therapeutics Res* 15(2):159-162.

Quebec Task Force on Spinal Disorders. 1987. Scientific approach to the assessment and management of activity-related spinal disorders. *Spine* 12:Suppl 1.

Quinn C, Chandler C, Moraska A. 2002. Massage therapy and frequency of chronic tension headaches. *Am J Public Health* 92:1657-1661.

Rattray FS, Ludwig L, Beglin G. 2000. *Clinical Massage Therapy: Understanding, Assessing and Treating Over 70 Conditions*. Toronto:Talus Inc.

Rexilius SJ, Mundt C, Erickson C, Megel M, Agrawal S. 2002. Therapeutic effects of massage therapy and handling touch on caregivers of patients undergoing autologous hematopoietic stem cell transplant. *Oncol Nurs Forum* 29:E35-44.

Richards KC. 1998. The effect of a back massage and relaxation intervention on sleep in critically ill patients. *Am J Crit Care* 7:288-299.

Rodenburg JB, Steenbeek P, Schiereck P, Bar PR. 1994. Warm-up, stretching and massage diminish harmful effects of eccentric exercise. *Int J Sports Med* 15:414-419

Rowe M, Alfred D. 1999. The effectiveness of slow-stroke massage in diffusing agitated behaviors in individuals with Alzheimer's disease. *J Gerontol Nurs* 25:22-34.

Sabri S, Roberts VC, Cotton LT. 1971. Prevention of early deep vein thrombosis by intermittent compression of the leg during surgery. *BMJ* 4:394.

Scafidi F & Field T. 1997. Massage therapy improves behavior in neonates born to HIV positive mothers. *J Ped Psychol* 21:889-897.

Scafidi F, Field T, Schanberg S, Bauer C, Vega-Lahr N, Garcia R. 1986. Effects of tactile/kinesthetic stimulation on the clinical course and sleep/wake behavior of preterm neonates. *Infant Behav Dev* 9:91-105.

Scafidi F, Field T, Wheeden A, Schanberg S, Kuhn C, Symanski R, Zimmerman E, Bandstra ES. 1996. Cocaine exposed preterm neonates show behavioral and hormonal differences. *Pediatrics* 97:851-855.

Schwellnus MP, Mackintosh L, Mee J. 1992. Deep transverse frictions in the treatment of iliotibial band friction syndrome in athletes: a clinical trial. *Physiotherapy* 78:564-568.

Scull CW. 1945. Massage - physiological basis. *Arch Phys Med* 26:159-167.

Severini V, Venerando A. 1967a. Effect on the peripheral circulation of substances producing hyperemia in combination with massage. *Europa Medicophys* 3:184-198.

Severini V, Venerando A. 1967b. The physiological effects of massage on the cardiovascular system. *Europa Medicophys* 3:165-183.

Shulman KR, Jones GE. 1996. The effectiveness of massage therapy intervention on reducing anxiety in the workplace. *J App Behav Sci* 32:160-173.

Simkin PP, O'Hara M. 2002. Nonpharmacologic relief of pain during labor: systematic reviews of five methods. *Am J Obstet Gynecol* 186:S131-159.

Simons DJ, Day E, Goodell H, Wolff HG. 1948. Cited in Jacobs, 1960. Experimental studies on headache: muscles of the scalp and neck as sources of pain. *Res Publ Assoc Res Nerv Ment Dis* 23:228-244.

Simpson J. 1991. Massage. Positive strokes in palliative care. *N Zeal Nurs J* July:15-17.

Sims S. 1986. Slow stroke back massage for cancer patients. *Nurs Times* 82:47-50.

Smith LL, Keating MN, Holbert D, Spratt DJ, McCammon MR, Smith SS, Israel RG. 1994. The effects of athletic massage on delayed onset muscle soreness, creatine kinase, and neutrophil count: a preliminary report. *JOSPT* 19(2):93-99.

Smith MC, Kemp J, Hemphill L, Vojir CP. 2002. Outcome of therapeutic massage for hospitalized cancer patients. *J Nurs Schol* 34:257-262.

SPORTS. 1986a. Recovery, Part 2. Overtraining. August: Adapted from Harre D (ed). *Principles of Sport Training*. Berlin: Sportverlag.

SPORTS. 1986b. Regeneration alternatives in high performance sport. February: Adapted from Das Betreuungssystem im Modernen Hochleitungssport. *Deutscher Sportbund, Bundesausschuss Leistungssport*.

St.-Pierre D, Gardiner PF. 1987. The effect of immobilization and exercise on muscle function: a review. *Physiother Can* 39:24-36.

Stamford, B. 1986. What are muscle cramps? *Physician Sportsmed* 14:192.

Starling EH. 1894. The influence of mechanical factors on lymph production. *J Physiol* 16:224-267.

Stephenson NL, Weinrich SP, Tavakoli AS. 2000. The effects of foot reflexology on anxiety and pain in patients with breast and lung cancer. *Oncol Nurs Forum* 27:67-72.

Sullivan SJ, Williams LRT, Seaborne DE, Morelli M. 1991. Effects of massage on alpha-motoneuron excitability. *Phys Ther* 71(8):555-560.

Sunshine W, Field T, Quintino O, Fierro K, Kuhn C, Burman I, Schanberg S. 1996. Fibromyalgia benefits from massage therapy and transcutaneous electrical stimulation. *J Clin Rheum* 2(1):18-22.

Suskind MI, Hajek NA, Hines HM. 1946. Effects of massage on denervated skeletal muscle. *Arch Phys Med* 27:133-135.

Swezey RL. 1983. The modern thrust of manipulation and traction therapy. *Semin Arthritis Rheum* 12:322-331.

Tappan FM, Benjamin PJ. 1998. *Tappan's Handbook of Healing Massage Techniques*, 3rd edition, Stamford CT, Appleton & Lange.

Taylor AG, Galper DI, Taylor P, Rice LW, Andersen W, Irwin W, Wang XQ, Harrell FE Jr. 2003. Effects of adjunctive Swedish massage and vibration therapy on short-term postoperative outcomes: a randomized controlled trial. *J Altern Complement Med* 9:77-89.

Tiidus PM, Shoemaker JK. 1995. Effleurage massage, muscle blood flow and long-term post-exercise strength recovery. *Int J Sports Med* 16:478-483

Travell JG, Simons DG. 1983. *Myofascial Pain and Dysfunction: The Trigger Point Manual*. Baltimore: Williams & Wilkins.

Trettin H. 1993. Schadel-hirn-traumen durch sport. *Lymphologie* 17:36-40.

Tucker E, Krueger S, Mooney E. 1998. A study on the effects of manual lymph drainage on fibromyalgia. *JSTM* Spring:8-12.

Urba SG. 1996. Nonpharmacologic pain management in terminal care. *Clin Geriatr Med* 12:301-311.

Valtonen EJ. 1967. Syncardial massage for treating extremities swollen by traumata, vein diseases or idiopathic lymphoedema. *Acta Chir Scand* 133:363-367.

Valtonen EJ, Lilius HG, Svinhufvud U. 1973. The effect of syncardial massage produced without synchronization and with different pressure impulse frequencies. *Ann Chir Gynaecol Fenn* 62:69-72.

van den Dolder PA, Roberts DL. 2003. A trial into the effectiveness of soft-tissue massage in the treatment of shoulder pain. *Aust J Physiother* 49:183-188.

Viitasalo JT, Niemela K, Kaappola R, Korjus T, Levola M, Mononen HV, Rusko HK, Takala TES. 1995. Warm underwater water-jet massage improves recovery from intense physical exercise. *Eur J Appl Physiol* 71:431-438.

Vodder E. 1965. Lymphdrainage. *Aesthet Med* 14:6.

Wakim KG, Martin GM, Terrier JC, Elkins EC, Krusen FH. 1949. The effects of massage on the circulation in normal and paralyzed extremities. *Arch Phys Med* 30:135-144.

Wakim KG, Martin GM, Krusen FH. 1955. Influence of centripetal rhythmic compression on localized edema of an extremity. *Arch Phys Med* 36:98.

Wakim KG. 1976. Chapter 2. Physiologic effects of massage. In Licht S, ed. *Massage, Manipulation and Traction*. Huntington, NY: Robert E. Krieger.

Wale JO. 1968. *Tidy's Massage and Remedial Exercises*. Bristol: John Wright & Sons.

Watson J. 1981a. Pain mechanisms: a review. I. Characteristics of peripheral receptors. *Aust J Physiother* 27:135-143.

Watson J. 1981b. Pain mechanisms: a review. II. Afferent pain pathways. *Aust J Physiother* 27:191-198.

Waylonis GW. 1967. Physiologic effects of ice massage. *Arch Phys Med Rehab* 48:37-42.

Weeks J. 2001. Post-legislative mandate: two-thirds of group health clinician respondents view CAM as effective. *The Integrator for the Bus of Alt Med* April, 2001.

Weiss JM. 1998. Treatment of leg edema and wounds in a patient with severe musculoskeletal injuries. *Phys Ther* 78:1104-1113.

Wheeden A, Scafidi FA, Field T, Ironson G, Valdeon C, Bandstra E. 1993. Massage effects on cocaine-exposed preterm neonates. *J Dev Behav Ped* 14:318-322.

Wiktorsson-Moller M, Oberg B, Ekstrand J, Gillquist J. 1983. Effects of warming up, massage, and stretching on range of motion and muscle strength in the lower extremity. *Am J Sports Med* 11:249-252.

Wilkie DJ, Kampbell J, Cutshall S, Halabisky H, Harmon H, Johnson LP, Weinacht L, Rake-Marona M. 2000. Effects of massage on pain intensity, analgesics and quality of life in patients with cancer pain: a pilot study of a randomized clinical trial conducted within hospice care delivery. *Hospice J* 15:31-53.

Wilkins RW, Halperin MH, Litter J. 1950. The effects of various physical procedures on circulation in human limbs. *Ann Intern Med* 33:1232-1245.

Williams AF, Vadgama A, Franks PJ, Mortimer PS. 2002. A randomized controlled crossover study of manual lymphatic drainage therapy in women with breast cancer-related lymphoedema. *Eur J Cancer Care* 11:254-261.

Witt PL, MacKinnon J. 1986. Trager psychophysical integration. A method to improve chest mobility of patients with chronic lung disease. *Phys Ther* 66:214-217.

Wolf SL. 1975. Skin analgesia and ice massage [letter]. *Phys Ther* 55:536.

Wolfson KJ. 1931. Studies on effect of physical therapeutic procedures on function and structure. *JAMA* 96:2019.

Wolsko PM, Eisenberg DM, Davis RB, Kessler R, Phillips RS. 2003. Patterns and perceptions of care for treatment of back and neck pain. *Spine* 28:292-297.

Wood EC, Becker PD. 1981. Effects of massage. In *Beard's Massage*. 3rd ed. Philadelphia: W.B. Saunders. pp 23-36.

Woodman RM, Pare L. 1982. Evaluation and treatment of soft tissue lesions of the ankle and forefoot using the Cyriax approach. *Phys Ther* 62:1144-1147.

Yackzan L, Adams C, Francis KT. 1984. The effects of ice massage on delayed muscle soreness. *Am J Sports Med* 12:159-165.

Yamazaki Z, Fujimori Y, Wada T, Togawa T, Yamakoshi K, Shimazu H. 1979. Admittance plethysmographic evaluation of undulatory massage for the edematous limb. *Lymphology* 12:40-42.

Yamazaki Z, Idezuki Y, Nemoto T, Togawa T. 1988. Clinical experiences using pneumatic massage therapy for edematous limbs over the last 10 years. *Angiology* 39:154-163.

Yoffey JM, Courtice FM. 1956. *Lymphatics, Lymph and Lymphoid Tissue: Their Physiological and Clinical Significance*. 2nd ed. London: Arnold.

Zanolla R, Monzeglio C, Balzarini A, Martino G. 1984. Evaluation of the results of three different methods of postmastectomy lymphedema treatment. *J Surg Oncol* 26:210-213.

Zeitlin D; Keller SE; Shiflett SC; Schleifer SJ; Bartlett JA. 2000. Immunological effects of massage therapy during acute academic stress. *Psychosom Med* 62:83-84.

INDEX

Page references in italics indicate an illustration. Page references followed by an italic *f* indicate a figure; those followed by an italic *t* indicate a table.